How Selegiline ((-)-Deprenyl) Slows Brain Aging

Authored By

Joseph Knoll

Semmelweis University
Department of Pharmacology and Pharmacotherapy
Budapest
Hungary

CONTENTS

CHAPTERS

FOREWORD

This is a most impressive work, a tour de force, by one of the pioneers of neuropsychopharmacology. It documents Joseph Knoll's research over six decades that led to the development of the first drug that could prolong longevity in several species of animals.

The story begins in the 1950s in the laboratories of the pharmacology department, Medical University of Budapest, where Knoll, while still a medical student, develops a methodology for the study of "acquired drives" (conditional reflexes) in rats.

Knoll's research continued in the 1960s with structure-activity studies of centrally acting stimulant drugs, in the course of which he discovered that one of the long-acting phenylethylamine derivatives, (-)-deprenyl, a substance with monoamine oxidase (MAO) inhibiting property, differed from all other MAO inhibitors available at the time by inhibiting the effects of tyramine. The discovery led to the introduction of (-)-deprenyl, referred to also as selegiline, into the treatment of depression as the first MAO-inhibitor without the cheese effect.

Instrumental to further development was Knoll's demonstration in 1970 that selegiline differed also from all other MAOIs available at the time by selectively inhibiting MAO-B, the enzyme involved in the oxidative deamination of dopamine. It led to the extension of selegiline's indications to Parkinsonism.

The turning point in Knoll's research with selegiline was his discovery in the 1980s that the drug enhanced catecholaminergic activity in doses much below that required for MAO inhibition. Important also was his demonstration that the age related decrease of dopamine content in the striatum and decline in sexual activity could be delayed by preventive treatment with the drug. These findings opened up the line of research that led to the demonstration that selegiline could prolong longevity in several species of animals by slowing "brain aging", as shown by the decrease in some age related changes, *e.g.*, accumulation of lipofuscin in brain cells.

The finding that some of the clinical effects of selegiline can be attributed to the enhancement of catecholaminergic activity, also opened up a new area of research in neuropharmacology: the screening for "enhancer" substances. One of the major contributions of this new area of research is Knoll's discovery of (-)-BPAP, a tryptamine derived enhancer of both serotonergic and catecholaminergic activity.

Knoll, a vigorous octogenarian, who has himself taken deprenyl for the past twenty years, is still fully active in his research. He is one of the last giants of a bygone era in pharmacology whose research was guided by theories. By using his theory of "enhancer regulation", as framework for presenting experiments conducted over years, Knoll makes it possible for readers to follow not only his findings but also his thinking. One wonders if he had operated without his theory whether some of the potential benefits of selegiline would have remained hidden.

Thomas A. Ban

Emeritus Professor of Psychiatry
Vanderbilt University
USA

PREFACE

Deprenyl, developed in the early 1960s with the aim to combine the psychostimulant effect of PEA with the psychoenergetic effect of the MAO inhibitors, became world-wide known and used as the first selective inhibitor of B-type MAO, which did not block the activity of the intestinal A-type MAO, thus was free from the cheese-effect.

Further studies revealed that in low doses, which leave MAO activity unchanged, deprenyl is enhancing, via a previously unknown mechanism, the activity of the catecholaminergic neurons in the brain stem and this catecholaminergic activity enhancer (CAE) effect is the primarily important pharmacological effect of deprenyl.

The main aim of this book, which recapitulates a part of information included in my previously published monograph „The Brain and Its Self" (Springer, 2005), is to focus attention to the theoretical and practical importance to the enhancer-regulation in the brain. It summarizes experimental and clinical data in support to the proposal that the prophylactic administration of a CAE substance during postdevelopmental life could significantly slow the aging-related decay of behavioral performances, prolong life, and prevent or delay the onset of aging-related neurodegenerative diseases such as Parkinson's and Alzheimer's. E-250, later named deprenyl, was one of the newly synthetized compounds in a structure-activity-relationship study which we performed in the early 1960s with the aim to combine the psychostimulant effect of PEA with the psychoenergetic effect of the MAO inhibitors.

There is no conflict of interest regarding the data in this book.

Joseph Knoll
Semmelweis University
Department of Pharmacology and Pharmacotherapy
Budapest
Hungary
jozsefknoll@hotmail.com

ABBREVIATIONS

Aβ(1-42)	:	amyloid-β-protein, Abeta protein
Aβ(25-35)	:	amyloid-β-protein fraction
ACh	:	acetylcholine
AD	:	Alzheimer's disease
AF64-A	:	methyl-β-acetoxyethyl-2-chloroethylamine
APOE	:	apolipoprotein E
BDNF	:	brain-derived neurotrophic factor
(-)-BPAP	:	R-(-)-1-(benzofuran-2-yl)-2-propylaminopentane
CAE effect	:	catecholaminergic activity enhancer effect
CAR	:	conditioned avoidance response
CNS	:	central nervous system
CDS	:	cognitive dysfunction syndrome
CR	:	conditioned reflex
CS	:	conditioned stimulus
DATATOP	:	Deprenyl And Tocopherol Antioxidant Therapy Of Parkinsonism
DSM-IV-TR	:	Diagnostic and Statistical Manual of Mental Disorders
DSP-4	:	N-(2-chloroethyl)-N-ethyl-2-bromobenzylamine
ECR	:	extinguishable conditioned reflex

EF	: escape failure
GABA	: γ-aminobutyric acid
GDNF	: glial cell-derived neurotrophic factor
GPRC	: G protein-coupled receptor
ICD-10	: International Statistical Classification of Diseases and Related Health Problems
ICR	: inextinguishable conditioned reflex
IR	: intertrial response
MAO	: monoamine oxidase
MAO-A	: A-type monoamine oxidase
MAO-B	: B-type monoamine oxidase
MDD	: major depressive disorder
$MPDP^+$	: 1-methyl-4-phenyl-2,3-dihydropyridinium ion
MPP^+	: methyl-phenyl-tetrahydro-pyridinium ion
MPTP	: 1-methyl-4-phenyl-1,2,3,6-tetrahydropyridine
NGF	: nerve growth factor
6-OHDA	: 6-hydroxydopamine
PEA	: β-phenylethylamine
PD	: Parkinson's disease
(-)-PPAP	: (-)-1-phenyl-2-propylaminopentane

SOD   : superoxide-dismutase

SSRI   : selective serotonin reuptake inhibitor

STS   : selegiline transmembrane system

TLS   : technical lifespan

TLS_h : human technical lifespan

TA   : trace amine

US   : unconditioned stimulus

KEYWORDS

Aging

Alzheimer's disease (AD)

Anti-aging drugs

(-)-BPAP: R-(-)-1-(benzofuran-2-yl)-2-propylaminopentane

Catecholaminergic activity enhancer (CAE) effect

DATATOP: Deprenyl And Tocopherol Antioxidant Therapy Of Parkinsonism

(-)-Deprenyl: (R)-N-methyl-N-(1-phenylpropan-2-yl)prop-2-yn-1-amine,

E-250, Selegiline, Eldepryl, Jumex, Emsam, Zelepar

Enhancer-regulation

Enhancer substances

-Natural: PEA, tryptamine

-Synthetic: (-)-deprenyl, (-)-PPAP, (-)-BPAP

Enhancer-sensitive neurons: catecholaminergic, serotonergic, hippocampal

Enhancer-sensitive cells: PC12, human brain capillary endothelial cells, mouse embrionic stem cell, murine embryonal carcinoma stem cell

Lifespan

Prolongation of lifespan

Longevity studies

Major depressive disorder (MDD)

Monoamine oxidase (MAO): A-type, B-type

Monoamine oxidase inhibitors: A-type, B-type

Neurotrophic factors

Parkinson's disease (PD)

PEA: β-phenylethylamine

(-)-PPAP: (-)-1-phenyl-2-propylaminopentane

INTRODUCTION

Memories of the Theoretical Foundation of my 60 Years in Research with Special Regard to the Development of (-)-Deprenyl/Selegiline

At the end of my third year in university, after my examination in pharmacology in February 1949, Professor Béla Issekutz Sen., chairman of the Department of Pharmacology of the Medical University (now Semmelweis University, Department of Pharmacology and Pharmacotherapy) in Budapest, invited me to join a research group in the Institute. I fell in love with brain research and worked day and night with my rats; I never left my lab for longer than a one month period in my life. From 1962 until 1992 I succeeded Béla Issekutz as head of the department where I am still working as a Professor Emeritus.

*

It is a horrifying fact that in Germany millions of single-minded little-men who had previously lived an honest simple life and never belonged to extremist groups, dramatically changed within a few years after 1933. Imbued with the Nazi ideology, they became unbelievably cool-headed murderers of innocent civilians during the Second World War. This phenomenon has been documented from many angles in dozens of novels, films, and so on. However, we are still waiting for an adequate elucidation of the brain mechanism responsible for this dramatic and rapid change in the behavior of millions.

As a survivor of Auschwitz and the Dachau death train (Dunn, 1998, pp. 209-211) I had the opportunity to directly experience a few typical representatives of this type of manipulated human beings, and I have had more than enough time and direct experience to reflect upon the essential changes in the physiological manipulability of the human brain. It was, therefore, probably not just by mere chance that when I started my behavioral studies in the early 1950s and discovered the ability of rats to acquire an unnatural drive, that I soon realized that this cortical mechanism may explain the manipulability of more sophisticated mammalian organisms. I succeeded in developing a rat model to study the nature of an acquired drive following the changes in the brain in the course of the acquisition of this drive from the start of training until its firm manifestation. Two enthusiastic students, Károly Kelemen and Berta Knoll, now distinguished scientists, joined me in this work.

We built a special acquired urge, the 'glass-cylinder-seeking drive', into the brain of rats (Knoll *et al.*, 1955 a,b,c, 1956; Knoll, 1956, 1957; see also Knoll, 1969, for review). Based on an unconditioned avoidance reflex (escape from a hot plate) and using the sound of a shrill bell, to play the role of a high-priority conditioned stimulus, rats were trained to search passionately for a 30-cm-high glass-cylinder and jump to the rim of it. The cylinder was open at bottom and top with diameters of 16 cm and 12 cm, respectively, and with a side opening through which a rat (up to 350-400 g body weight) could manage to get inside the cylinder.

In the training procedure the rat was pushed through the side opening of the glass-cylinder standing on a metal plate heated to 60°C, and the jumping reflex was elicited for a couple of weeks three times daily on 10-50 occasions at 10s intervals with bell and heat stimulation. After a short training period a chain of inextinguishable conditioned reflexes (ICRs) developed and the rat indefatigably displayed the jumping reflex without heat stimulation, even 100 times in succession (Knoll *et al.*, 1955 a,b,c). This was a transient stage leading to the manifestation of the glass-cylinder-seeking drive (for review see Knoll, 1969; Chapter 4).

The rats that performed best in this study acquired the glass-cylinder-seeking drive in a stable manner, thereafter maintaining this unnatural urge for a lifetime. The rats showed the same high-grade adaptability and readiness in overcoming different obstacles during goal-attainment as the ones influenced by innate drives, such as hunger or sexual desire (Knoll *et al.*, 1956; Knoll, 1956, 1957). In the most efficiently trained, best performing rats, the acquired drive was so powerful that it prevailed over life's most important innate drives. When such a rat has been deprived of food for 48 hours and then food was offered within the usual setup that contained the glass-cylinder, the rat looked for the glass-cylinder, and left the food untouched. Similarly, when a receptive female was offered to a fully sexually active glass-cylinder-seeking male rat in the usual setup, the male looked for the glass-cylinder and neglected the receptive female. The mouse, a rodent closely related to the rat, trained under the same experimental conditions as the rat, was unable to acquire the glass-cylinder-seeking drive (Berta Knoll 1961, 1968). Thus, it was a reasonable conclusion that vertebrates can be divided into three groups according to the mode of operation of their brain: (a) those that operate with innate drives only (the majority); (b) those with an ability to acquire drives (a minority); and (c) the 'group of one' that operates almost exclusively with acquired drives (*Homo sapiens*).

With the evolution of brains capable of acquiring drives, species appeared whose members could manipulate each other's behavior and act in concert. This was the condition *sine qua non* for the evolution of social living, a form of life that enabled the species to surpass qualitatively the performance of any given individual. It goes without saying that training members in the skills needed to act in concert improved the quality of life. The learned behavior, for example, of five to six hungry female lions acting in unison to separate from the herd the animal chosen to be brought down, significantly increases the chance of capturing the prey. It was the evolution of the brain with the ability to acquire drives that made the appearance of life on earth so immensely variable.

With the development of the human brain, a functional network with over 100 billion interrelated nerve cells and 10^{11} bit capacity arose. With this system, whose operation is inseparably connected to conscious perception, life on earth reached its most sophisticated form. Furthermore, the human being, who is primarily a social creature, is a building block in the creation of a gigantic product: human society. The function and capacity of society obviously exceeds the sum of the activity of its members. Based on the practically inexhaustible capacity of the human brain to acquire drives, the human society represents a qualitatively new, higher form of life. For example, a country, presently the most sophisticated form of a human community, consists of millions or even over a billion humans and operates *de facto* as a huge living complex interacting with other similar entities, about 200 at present.

The birth and development of the human society, a moment insignificant and fleeting in the endless history of the universe, necessarily means everything to us.

It can be taken for granted that at the birth of human society, probably somewhere in South-Africa, very small groups formed a micro-community, working together. Due to learning, practice, and experience, their community life became more and more efficient, and the accumulation of basic knowledge opened the way for a more rapid development, truly reflected in population growth.

In the last phase of the Stone Age, about 8,000-9,000 years before our age, marked by the domestication of animals, development of agriculture, and the manufacture of pottery and textile, the human population on earth approached the *one million* level. Thereafter, however, the population increase went from strength to strength. By the beginning of the Common Era it had reached the *300 million* level, grew to *1.6 billion* to 1900, and is at present around *7 billion.*

A detailed analysis of the course of events until the rat acquired the glass-cylinder-seeking drive inspires the conclusion that *in the mammalian brain capable to acquire drives, untrained cortical neurons (Group 1) possess the potentiality to change their functional state in response to practice, training, or experience in three consecutive stages, namely getting involved either (i) in an extinguishable conditioned reflex (ECR) (Group 2); or (ii) in an inextinguishable conditioned reflex (ICR) (Group 3); or (iii) in an acquired drive (Group 4).* The study (Kelemen *et al.*, 1961) performed in Daniel Bovet's famous department in Rome by Károly Kelemen in Vincenzo G. Longo's laboratory, which presented experimental evidence for the expected *qualitative* difference in the EEG arousal reaction in extinguishable and non-extinguishable conditioned reflexes, accelarated the development of my theory.

All in all, it seems reasonable to conclude that the ability to acquire an irrepressible urge for a goal that is not necessary for survival was the last step in the development of the mammalian brain. This is the most sophisticated function of the telencephalon.

By the end of 1953, my experiments with the glass-cylinder seeking rats strongly urged me to shape the working hypothesis that the appearance of the mammalian brain with the ability to acquire drives produced species fit for domestic life, *i.e.* to live in intimate association with and to the advantage of humans. This ability of the mammalian brain ensured the interaction of the individual and the group, and finally led to the evolution of the most sophisticated form of organized life, the human society. After 16-years of research, I formulated my theory regarding the *peculiar role of the acquired drives in the evolution of mammalian life* in a monograph (Knoll, 1969).

To develop the full possibilities of this approach, I tried thereafter to clarify during a 36-year research period those key important brain mechanisms which determine the life of mammalian species whose members, being capable or fixing acquired drives, possess a brain with a higher level of manipulability than mammalian species whose cortex is missing this potential. I finally summarized my theory *"The Brain and Its Self. A Neurochemical Concept of the Innate and Acquired Drives"* in a second monograph (Knoll, 2005). I considered to answer from a new angle the three fundamental questions of human beings: Where do we come from?, Who are we?, Where are we going?

The physiology of the acquired drives furnishes knowledge about the most important brain mechanism which created the society: the manipulability of the cortex. An acquired drive is always built on one of the inner drives that ensures the survival of the individual or the species. However, after the acquired drive has been ultimately fixed, its origin, the innate drive cannot be recognized anymore either in man or a domesticated animal. A glass-cylinder seeking rat will never acquire this drive under natural conditions. The experimenter consciously manipulated the rat's brain, making use of the innate potential to change a group of cortical neurons *via* proper training in a way that the rat is fixing an acquired drive. Finally, the glass-cylinder seeking rat behaves as one who has a 'fanatical' desire for the glass-cylinder. Essentially the same mechanism works in all mammals capable to acquire drives.

Humans possess the most manipulable brain among all living creatures on earth. The brain of a suicide killer is furtively manipulated. The properly acquired drive develops as a result of long-lasting training. The subject always acts under coercion, under severe mental pressure. Nevertheless, it is the nature of acquired drives that if the manipulation was fully successful the individual ultimately behaves as one possessing a fanatical desire to reach the acquired-drive-motivated goal.

The main message of my theory is that human society is still in the trial- and - error phase of its development. It already seeks to bring to an end the myths-directed era, the first part of its history, and reach its final goal: the rationally directed human society in which behavioral modification induced by the home/school/society triad will be based, from birth until death, on the exact knowledge of the natural laws that keep the brain and its self going. In this way, members of the community will be raised to understand how the human cortex created with its chaos function the myths of supernatural forces. This was the ideology which enabled to bring into existence the human society prior to the *sine qua non* knowledge of the creative and controlling forces in the universe needed to establish and maintain a rationally directed homogenous human society.

It seems to be evident that the power of thinking in orderly rational ways, *i.e.* the capacity to understand the natural world (science) is that physiological reality which determines the conscious fight of the individual to find and fix acquired drives that optimally fit their natural endowments. Since *Homo sapiens* appeared around 150,000 years ago; reached full behavioral modernity around 50,000 years ago, and piled up little by little proper knowledge regarding the natural forces, time is already ripe for the transition to a rationally directed global human society. Enlightenment, the separation of Church, by its nature the main creator and guardian force of the myths-directed era of the human society, and State, interested by its nature in supporting with passing time more and more the rationally directed human activities, was more than 200 years ago the decisive step which enhanced with a previously unimaginable rapidity the development of science and technology.

Nevertheless, the chaos in which at the present 7 billion humans now live together on earth is due to the heterogeneity of myths that shaped their lives during previous millennia. The ultimately unavoidable transition of human society from the myths-directed era into the rationally-directed one will finally lead to a reasonably and harmoniously operating global human world. The aim set by the brilliant pioneers of the Enlightenment, their prudence recommendation: *Sapere aude* (Dare to go independent), is as timely as it was then. If masses learn how the brain works, they will resist traditional methods of manipulation.

*

My behavioral studies compelled me to start in the early 1960s a structure-activity-relationship study aiming to find a better psychic energizer than amphetamine and methamphetamine. I used these compounds to stimulate the catecholaminergic machinery in the brain stem, the neuronal network which plays the key role in the activation of the cortex.

The problem with amphetamine and methamphetamine is that as soon as the dose surpasses the 1-2 mg/kg level, the drug-induced continuous, irresistible release of catecholamines from their intraneuronal stores in the brain stem neurons arrives to an intensity resulting in aimless hypermotility which blocks purposeful behavior. In the early 1960s, monoamine oxidase (MAO) inhibitors represented a new type of central stimulation, so I decided to start the structure-activity-relationship study with methamphetamine containing a propargyl-group attached to the nitrogen. This group was known to form a covalent binding with the flavin in MAO and block the enzyme irreversibly. Out of a series of newly synthesized patentable methamphetamine derivatives, E-250 (later named deprenyl) was selected as the most suitable. The first paper describing its beneficial pharmacological properties was published in 1964 (in Hungarian) and in 1965 (in English) and the (-) isomer ((-)-deprenyl (Selegiline)) was the developed drug (Knoll *et al.*, 1964, 1965).

(-)-Deprenyl, the β-phenylethylamine (PEA)-derivative which catalyzed the discovery of the *catecholaminergic activity enhancer (CAE) effect* and opened my mind to the key importance of the enhancer regulation in brain work, is now a worldwide used drug to treat Parkinson's disease (PD), Alzheimer's disease (AD) and major depression disease (MDD). (-)-Deprenyl was not only an experimental tool of significant value in the development of my theory, but it also played a major role in the birth and development of anti-aging research. Today, it is the only compound which can extend life even beyond the "technical lifespan" of a species.

Herman Blaschko, one of the great researchers of the monoamine field who first suggested that dopamine might possess a physiological role in its own right, explained in his "Introduction and Historical Background" of the Festschrift dedicated to him (Costa & Sandler, 1972) why monoamine oxidase (MAO), the enzyme which oxidizes catecholamines was described in 1928 by its discoverer,

Mary Hare, as a tyramine oxidase (Hare, 1928): "…tyramine, the first substrate of MAO to be described, had not then been convincingly shown to occur in mammals. Miss Hare tested adrenaline as a possible substrate, but met with no success. The oxidation of the catecholamines by MAO was only discovered after we had learned to exclude the so-called 'autoxidation' of adrenaline in aqueous solutions" (Blaschko *et al.*, 1937). Something similar happened to me when I developed (-)-deprenyl. Hidden traps often slow the recognition of essential conditions in research. We arrived in the mid-1990s to the final experimental evidence that (-)-deprenyl is primarily a CAE-substance, and it exerts this effect in much lower than the MAO-B inhibitory dose (Knoll *et al.*, 1996a,b,c).

Earlier, I was satisfied with the working hypothesis that the selective inhibition of MAO-B in the brain is fully responsible for the beneficial therapeutic effects of our compound. We were pleased that this view was generally accepted and (-)-deprenyl, the first selective inhibitor of MAO-B, became an important experimental tool in MAO research. On the other hand, since MAO inhibitors fell into disrepute because of the cheese-effect and (-)-deprenyl was free of the catecholamine releasing effect of its parent compounds (Knoll *et al.*, 1968), the new substance was of great promise from therapeutic point of view.

It was the period before the discovery that PEA and its long acting derivatives, amphetamine and methamphetamine, were primarily CAE substances. Now, it is already clear that the main physiological effect of PEA remained undetected because the catecholamine releasing property concealed its CAE effect. (-)-Deprenyl, the peculiar PEA-derivative, that is free of the catecholamine releasing property, provided us with the opportunity to study the operation of the enhancer regulation in catecholaminergic neurons in the brain stem and to understand that the CAE effect of PEA is of primary physiological importance.

Since the disciples and admirers of Herman Blaschko met at the first international symposium on MAO in Cagliari (Sardinia) in June, 1971, where I presented the first experimental evidence that (-)-deprenyl is a selective inhibitor of MAO-B, and met again in 1975 at the CIBA Symposium "Monoamine oxidase and its inhibitors" in London, where I presented the lecture "Analysis of the pharmacological effects of selective monoamine oxidase inhibitors" (Knoll,

1976), thousands of papers shed light on the chemical nature and physiological significance of the two forms of MAO. (-)-Deprenyl, played in this development a key role as an experimental tool. This is probably the reason why selegiline is since decades firmly treated as the classic selective inhibitor of MAO-B, and its CAE effect which deserves first and foremost attention failed, up to the present day, to become common knowledge.

It is the main aim of this book to piece facts and arguments together which all go to show that selegiline, due to its CAE effect, slows the aging-related decay of the catecholaminergic brain engine, and this is why the maintenance on a low daily dose of selegiline helps to maintain physical and mental vigor in the latter decades of life, and is also a chance to significantly decrease the prevalence of PD and AD. *To motivate clinicians to think the matter over inspired this work.*

How Selegiline ((-)-Deprenyl) Slows Brain Aging

2

Send Orders of Reprints at reprints@benthamscience.org

CHAPTER 1

(-)-Deprenyl(Selegiline), The First Selective Inhibitor of B-Type MAO and the Unique One Free of the Cheese Effect

The discovery of the MAO inhibitors in the early 1950s played a leading role in the birth of neuropsychopharmacology. The rapid development of this new, independent branch in brain science soon changed, in a revolutionary manner, the general views about the principals of behavior and radically altered human attitudes toward derangements in psychic function.

In the beginning there was a keen interest in the MAO inhibitors, of which a substantial number were developed and introduced into clinical practice, but because of serious side-effects there was a rapid turnover in the introduction and withdrawal of these drugs.

In 1963, in The Lancet, a calamitous number of clinical reports (Womack, Foster, Maan, Davies) gave account of the observation that patients treated with MAO inhibitors (tranylcypromine, nialamide, pargyline) developed temporally clinical symptoms (hypertension, palpitation, neck stiffness, headache, nausea, vomiting), similar to a paroxysm produced by pheochromocytoma. Blackwell suggested that the hypertensive crises are associated with the ingestion of high amounts of tyramine in cheese, the metabolism of which is inhibited by the MAO inhibitors ("cheese effect") (Blackwell, 1963). This conclusion was correct. Cheese and many other foods containing tyramine were found to provoke hypertensive episodes in patients treated with MAO inhibitors. The "cheese effect" restricted the clinical use of this group of drugs.

Deprenyl (we used the racemic compound under the code name E-250 in the first series of experiments) proved to be a compound with a peculiar pharmacological spectrum. The (-) enantiomer of E-250 (selegiline((-)-deprenyl)) was finally selected for therapeutic use. As the parent compound of (-)-methamphetamine, (-)-deprenyl is a long acting PEA-derivative which contains a propargyl group. This group in (-)-deprenyl makes a covalent binding preferentially with the flavin in B-type MAO, thus it blocks this type of MAO irreversibly. (-)-Deprenyl was first described as a highly potent and selective inhibitor of MAO-B, and is still primarily used as an experimental tool for this purpose. Fig. **1** shows the chemical structure of selegiline.

We described E-250 as a new spectrum psychic energizer (Knoll *et al.*, 1964, 1965). E-250 was selected for further development because I was fascinated by a surprisingly unexpected behavior of this compound. MAO inhibitors potentiate blood pressure which increases the effect of amphetamine, a releaser of norepinephrine from their stores in the noradrenergic nerve terminals. E-250 *inhibited* the pressor effect of amphetamine (see Fig. **1** in Knoll *et al.*, 1965). Based on this observation, we analyzed this peculiar behavior in more detail. As expected, the studies revealed that *deprenyl, in contrast to the known MAO inhibitors, did not potentiate the effect of tyramine but inhibited it.* This effect of deprenyl was first demonstrated in a study performed on cats and on the isolated vas deferens of rats. The hope was expressed in the discussion and summary of this paper that this peculiar tyramine-inhibiting property of a potent MAO inhibitor may be of special therapeutic value (Knoll *et al.*, 1968).

In the same year when we published the unique behavior of (-)-deprenyl, Johnston described a substance, later named clorgyline, that came into world-wide use as an experimental tool in MAO research (Johnston, 1968). He namely realized that clorgyline preferentially inhibits the deamination of serotonin, and this important finding was soon confirmed by Hall *et al.* (1969). Johnston proposed the existence of two forms of MAO, "type A" and "type B", the former being selectively inhibited by clorgyline and the latter relatively insensitive to it. Johnston's nomenclature has become widely accepted and is still in use. Clorgyline remained the classic selective inhibitor of A-type MAO.

For further studies a selective inhibitor of MAO-B was badly needed. I was lucky to realize that (-)-deprenyl was the missing, highly selective inhibitor of MAO-B and presented this finding in my lecture at the First International MAO Meeting in Cagliary (Sardinia) in 1971. (-)-Deprenyl was used thereafter as the specific experimental tool to analyze B-type MAO. The first paper which described this novel property (Knoll & Magyar, 1972) has become ten years later a citation classic (Knoll J, This Week's Citation Classic, January 15, 1982). For several years the selective MAO-B inhibitory effect was at the center of our interest. It delayed the discovery of the drug's enhancer effect. It was the MAO inhibitory effect of the compound that led to the first clinical application of (-)-deprenyl.

In light of the serious side effects of levodopa in PD, Birkmayer and Hornykiewicz tried to achieve a levodopa-sparing effect by the concurrent administration of levodopa with an MAO inhibitor. As such combinations frequently elicited hypertensive attacks, they were soon compelled to terminate this line of clinical research (Birkmayer & Hornykiewicz, 1962).

Since we demonstrated in animal experiments that (-)-deprenyl is the unique MAO inhibitor that instead to potentiate the catecholamine-releasing effect of indirectly acting amines, inhibits it, we proposed to use this compound as an MAO inhibitor free of the cheese effect (Knoll *et al.*, 1968). The validity of this proposal was tested in volunteers by Sandler and his co-workers. They confirmed that in harmony with our findings in animal experiments, (-)-deprenyl is in humans an MAO inhibitor free of the cheese effect (Elsworth *et al.*, 1978; Sandler *et al.*, 1978). Considering the peculiar pharmacological profile of (-)-deprenyl, Birkmayer was the first clinician who dared to combine (-)-deprenyl with levodopa in PD. The trial was successful. The levodopa-sparing effect was achieved in patients without signs of significant hypertensive reactions (Birkmayer *et al.*, 1977). This study initiated and a following Lancet Editorial (September 25, 1982) enhanced the world-wide use of (-)-deprenyl in PD.

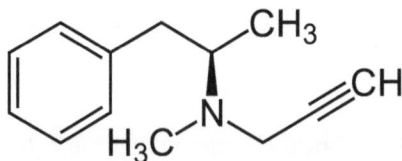

Systematic (IUPAC) name: (*R*)-*N*-methyl-*N*-(1-phenylpropan-2-yl)prop-2-yn-1-amine

Selegiline((-)-Deprenyl))

(Eldepryl, Jumex, Emsam, Zelepar)

Figure 1: The chemical structure of Selegiline((-)-Deprenyl) and the best known preparations in circulation.

CHAPTER 2

The Catecholaminergic Activity Enhancer Effect of (-)-Deprenyl and R-(-)-1-(Benzofuran-2-yl)-2-Propylaminopentane [(-)-BPAP]

The demonstration that multiple small dose administration of (-)-deprenyl enhances catecholaminergic activity in the brain and this effect is unrelated to MAO-B inhibition (Knoll & Miklya, 1994), catalyzed the discovery that (-)-deprenyl acts as a highly specific CAE substance (Knoll *et al.*, 1996a), and revealed the operation of the enhancer regulation in the catecholaminergic neurons in the brain stem. This finding clarified that PEA, the natural brain constituent, and the parent compound of deprenyl acts similarly and this is the main physiological effect of this important trace-amine (Knoll *et al.*, 1996c). To date, PEA, a highly potent releaser of catecholamines from their intraneuronal pools, is still classified as the prototype of the indirectly acting sympathomimetics. However, under natural conditions PEA acts as a selective CAE substance. From the very beginning the catecholamine-releasing effect of PEA was observed and studied in detail. The catecholamine releasing effect of PEA is exerted in much higher than the physiological concentrations of this trace-amine. This property of PEA completely concealed its CAE effect, which remained unidentified. (-)-Deprenyl, the unique PEA-derivative which is devoid of the catecholamine-releasing property, enabled me to realize that PEA acts under natural conditions in the brain as a highly selective CAE substance and (-)-deprenyl is a PEA-derived long-acting synthetic CAE substance (Knoll *et al.*, 1996a,c; Knoll, 1998).

It was the high pressure liquid chromatography (HPLC) method with electrochemical detection which allowed measuring exactly the amounts of catecholamines released continuously from freshly excised brain tissue that ensured to get unequivocal experimental evidence for the operation of the enhancer regulation in the life-important catecholaminergic and serotonergic system in the brain stem. We started in 1993 to measure with this technique the release of dopamine from the striatum, substantia nigra, and tuberculum olfactorium, the release of norepinephrine from the locus coeruleus, and the release of serotonin from the raphe.

We presented in 1994 the results of the first series of experiments performed with the HPLC method which demonstrated that multiple, small dose administration of (-)-deprenyl enhances catecholaminergic activity in the brain and this effect is unrelated to MAO-B inhibition (Knoll and Miklya, 1994).

We compared in this study the dose related enhancer effect of (-)-deprenyl, (-)-methamphetamine and (-)-1-phenyl-2-propylaminopentane [(-)-PPAP] on male and female rats, respectively. We treated daily the rats with the selected dose of the drugs for 21 days, removed the appropriate brain samples 24 hours after the last injection and measured the amount of the biogenic amines released from the tissue sample during 20 minutes. In both males and females treatment with (-)-deprenyl enhanced the release of dopamine from the striatum, substantia nigra and tuberculum olfactorium (significant in 0.01-0.25 mg/kg) and of noradrenaline from the locus coeruleus (significant in 0.05-0.25 mg/kg), whilst the release of serotonin from the raphe did not change in the rats treated with 0.01 - 0.25 mg/kg (-)-deprenyl.

Table **1** shows a few data demonstrating the priviously unknown enhancer effect of (-)-deprenyl, and (-)-PPAP, the (-)-deprenyl-analog devoid of the MAO inhibitory potency, and the finding that (-)-methamphetamine is a CAE substance in a dose as low as 0.05 mg/kg. The well known motility increasing effect of (-)-methamphetamine is undectable below 1 mg/kg. This early finding was in good agreement with our further results. *(-)-Deprenyl is a selective CAE substance.*

(-)-PPAP, the deprenyl-analog free of MAO inhibitory potency but otherwise possessing the same pharmacological spectrum as deprenyl (Knoll *et al.*, 1992a), acted essentially similarly to (-)-deprenyl. (-)-Methamphetamine, the parent compound of (-)-deprenyl, enhanced both dopminergic and noradrenergic activity, similarly to deprenyl. (-)-Methamphetamine diminished the serotonergic activity in both sexes.

The data presented in this study clearly proved that the daily administration of low doses of (-)-deprenyl, which leave MAO-B activity in the brain unchanged, keep the catecholaminergic neurons in the brain stem on a higher activity level and this specific CAE effect is detectable even 24 hours after the last injection of the drug.

We soon demonstrated that PEA and tyramine are mixed-acting sympathomimetic amines in the brain. They are primarily CAE substances and in much higher concentrations only releasers of the catecholamines from their intraneuronal pools (Knoll *et al.*, 1996 a). We further proved that (-)-deprenyl is a unique synthetic variant of PEA that is devoid of the catecholamine releasing property which concealed the detection of the CAE effect of PEA. Since (-)-deprenyl was the first PEA-derivative which did not release catecholamines from the interneuronal transmitter pools, it allowed to discover the operation of the enhancer regulation in the catecholaminergic brain stem neurons (Knoll *et al.*1996/b).

Table 1: Release of biogenic amines from brain samples of male and female rats, respectively, treated with the drugs daily for 21 days. (data taken from knoll and miklya, 1994)

Treatment MALES	Daily Dose (mg/kg)	Amount of Biogenic Amine (nmoles/g Tissue) Released from the Tissue Within 20 min				
		Dopamine			Norepinephrine	Serotonin
		Striatum	Substantia Nigra	Tuberculum Olfactorium	Locus Coeruleus	Raphe
Saline	-	2.72±0.10	2.96±0.13	2.58±0.56	4.10±0.18	0.461±0.01
(-)-Deprenyl	0.01	3.27±0.14***	4.17±0.31****	3.08±0.18***	6.13±0.62***	0.519±0.05
(-)-PPAP	0.10	5.17±0.29****	4.52±0.46****	5.2±0.21***	7.93±0.69****	0.466±0.03
(-)-Methamphetamine	0.05	3.77±0.08****	3.53±0.23*	3.65±0.19****	6.20±0.26****	0.214±0.02****
FEMALES						
Saline	-	2.42±0.06	2.80±0.03	2.42±0.10	3.67±0.23	0.460±0.03
(-)-Deprenyl	0.01	3.20±0.08***	3.18±0.07***	3.37±0.09***	3.97±0.23	0.444±0.02
	0.05	3.73±0.27***	3.55±0.19***	3.35±0.18***	7.70±0.10***	0.370±0.04
(-)-PPAP	0.10	4.90±0.26****	5.65±0.26****	5.02±0.21****	7.93±0.69****	0.390±0.01
(-)-Methamphetamine	0.05	2.87±0.14***	3.62±0.10****	2.85±0.11**	5.23±0.52***	0.300±0.04**

*P<0,05; **P<0,02; ***P<0,01; ****P<0,001;

Table **2** is summarizing the essential differences in the pharmacological spectrum of PEA and the amphetamines *versus* (-)-deprenyl and (-)-PPAP, the CAE substances devoid of the catecholamine-releasing property of their parent compounds. PEA, the natural brain constituent is in low concentration a CAE substance, in higher concentration a releaser of catecholamines from their interneuronal pools and a substrate to MAO, thus a rapidly metabolized, short acting agent. Amphetamine and methamphetamine act like PEA, but since they are not metabolized by MAO, they are long acting compounds. (-)-Deprenyl, the PEA-derivative free of the catecholamine-releasing property is a CAE substance and in much higher doses a selective inhibitor of MAO-B. (-)-PPAP acts like (-)-deprenyl, but is devoid of MAO inhibitory potency.

Table 2: Essential differences in the pharmacological spectrum of PEA and the amphetamines *versus* (-)-deprenyl and (-)-PPAP

CH_2-CH-N				Enhancer Effect	Releasing Effect	Relation to MAO
β-Phenylethylamine	H	H	H	+	+	MAO-B Substrate
Amphetamine	CH₃	H	H	+	+	Weak MAO Inhibitor
Methamphethamine	CH₃	CH₃	H	+	+	Weak MAO Inhibitor
(-)-1-Phenyl-2-Methyl-N-Methyl-Propargylamine, (-)-**Deprenyl**	CH₃	CH₃	C₃H₃	+	0	Selective MAO-B Inhibitor
(-)-1-Phenyl-2-Propylaminopenatane, (-)-**PPAP**	C₃H₇	H	C₃H₇	+	0	0

We can define enhancer regulation as: the existence of enhancer-sensitive neurons capable of changing their excitability in a split second and working on a higher activity level, due to endogenous enhancer substances. Of the natural brain constituents with such effect, for the time being, only PEA and tryptamine have been experimentally analyzed (Knoll, 2001, 2003, 2005).

The catecholaminergic and serotonergic neurons in the brain stem are excellent models to study the enhancer regulation since they supply the brain continuously with proper amounts of monoamines that influence practically all behavioral functions. The significant enhancement of the nerve-stimulation-induced release of [³H]-norepinephrine, [³H]-dopamine, and [³H]-serotonin from the isolated brain stem of the rat in the presence of PEA or tryptamine (Figs. **2,3,4**) is shown to illustrate the response of enhancer-sensitive brain stem neurons to endogenous enhancer substances.

To date we have studied in detail the enhancer effect of two natural brain constituents, PEA and tryptamine. From a freshly isolated brain stem of a pretreated rat a low amount of the labeled transmitters is released for a couple of hours (see Knoll & Miklya, 1995 for methodology). Neurons respond to stimulation in an "all or none" manner. The calculated average amount of each of the transmitters released from the non-stimulated brain stem is the product of the spontaneous firing of the most excitable, most responsive group of neurons of the surviving population with large individual variation in excitability. The overwhelming majority of the neurons remain silent. Electrical stimulation excites a further group of neurons as shown by the significant increase of the outflow of transmitters. Natural enhancer substances increase specifically the excitability of the enhancer-sensitive neurons. They enhance the impulse propagation mediated release of norepinephrine, dopamine and serotonin, and in the presence of PEA or tryptamine we observed the significantly enhanced release of [^{3}H]-norepinephrine (Fig. **2**), [^{3}H]-dopamine (Fig. **3**), and [^{3}H]-serotonin (Fig. **4**) to electrical stimulation.

Since a lower concentration of tryptamine (1.3 µmol/l) proved to be much more potent in enhancing the stimulation-evoked release of serotonin than a much higher concentration of PEA (16 µmol/l), this indicates that, on a molecular level, the enhancer regulation in the catecholaminergic and serotonergic neurons are not identical. Enhancer regulation in the brain heralds a new line of research. It brings different perspective to the brain-organized goal-oriented behavior since it seems to represent the device in the mammalian brain that operates as the *vis vitalis*.

All in all, PEA and amphetamines, the long-acting PEA-derivatives, are CAE substances which in higher concentrations release catecholamines from their intraneuronal stores, and *(-)-deprenyl is the unique PEA-derived synthetic CAE substance devoid of catecholamine releasing property.*

A comparison of the release of [^{3}H]-norepinephrine from isolated rat brain stem in the presence of (-)-amphetamine (Fig. **5**) and (-)-deprenyl (Fig. **7**) illustrates the essential difference in the pharmacological profile between the two synthetic PEA-derivatives. (-)-Amphetamine is a releaser of norepinephrine and (-)-deprenyl is devoid of this property. Fig. **5** shows that in the presence of

(-)-amphetamine, norepinephrine is continuously released and the electrical stimulation of the brain stem is unable to release further amounts of the transmitter. Thus the catecholamine-releasing effect of (-)-amphetamine conceals the detectability of the CAE effect of this long-acting synthetic PEA-derivative. Fig. **6** shows that after repeated electrical stimulations, due to exhaustion, the amount of [^{3}H]-norepinephrine released from an isolated rat brain is on a slow continuous decline. Fig. **7** shows that (-)-deprenyl, devoid of the catecholamine-releasing property, makes the CAE effect clearly visible. Fig. **8** demonstrates that (-)-deprenyl is capable of enhancing in an extremely low, 0.2 picog/ml, concentration the release of ^{3}[H]-dopamine from the isolated rat brain stem to electrical stimulation.

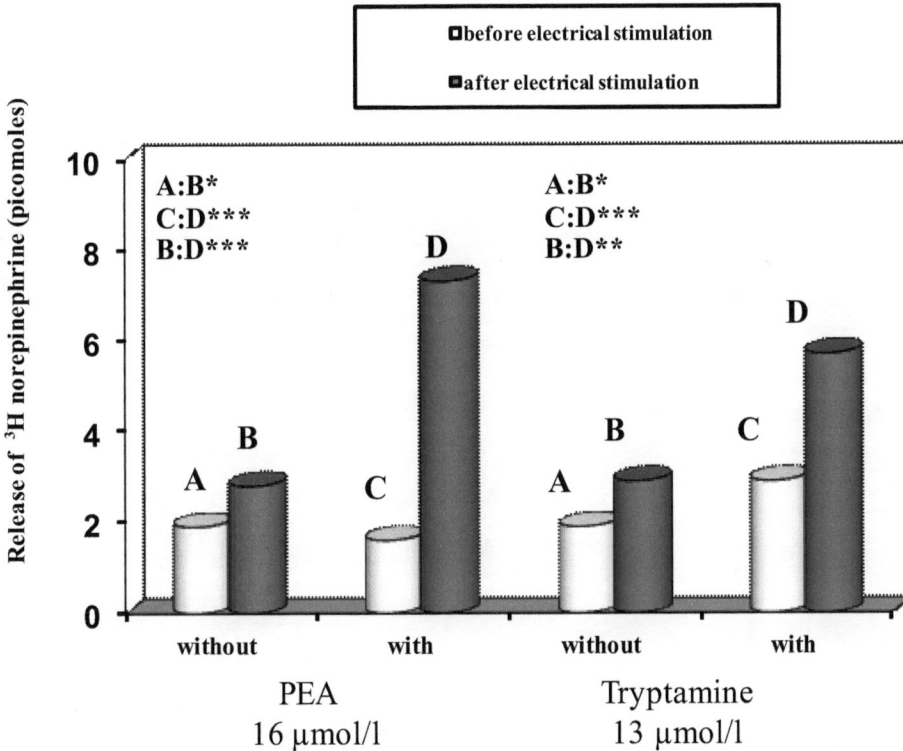

Figure 2: Significant enhancement of the nerve-stimulation-induced release of [^{3}H]-norepinephrine from the isolated brain stem of the rat in the presence of β-phenylethylamine (PEA) and tryptamine, respectively (N=8). Each graph bar represents the amount of the labeled transmitter in picomoles released in a 3-min collection period. See Knoll *et al.* (1996c) for methodology. Paired Student's *t*-test was used for statistical analysis. *P<0.05, **P<0.02, ***P<0.001.

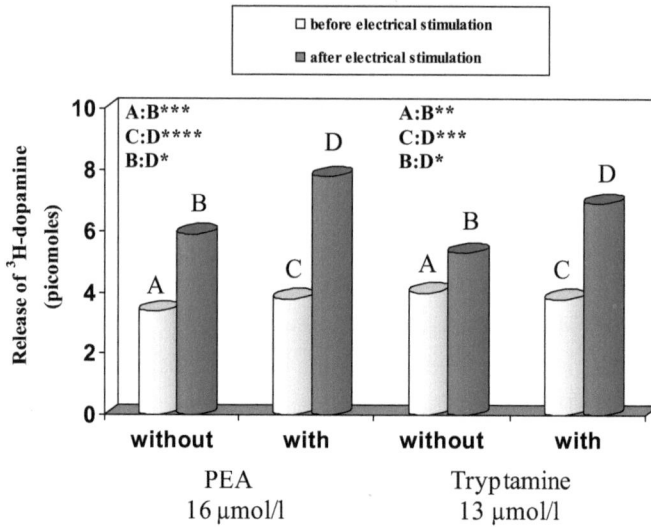

Figure 3: Significant enhancement of the nerve-stimulation-induced release of [³H]-dopamine from the isolated brain stem of the rat in the presence of β-phenylethylamine (PEA) and tryptamine, respectively (N=8). Each graph bar represents the amount of the labeled transmitter in picomoles released in a 3-min collection period. See Knoll *et al.* (1996c) for methodology. Paired Student's *t*-test was used for statistical analysis. *$P<0.05$, **$P<0.02$, ***$P<0.01$, ****$P<0.001$.

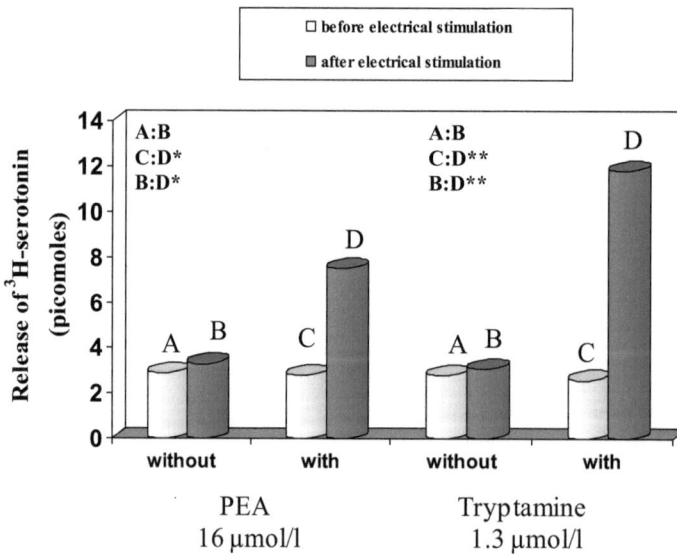

Figure 4: Significant enhancement of the nerve-stimulation-induced release of [³H]-serotonin from the isolated brain stem of the rat in the presence of β-phenylethylamine (PEA) and tryptamine, respectively (N=8). Each graph bar represents the amount of the labeled transmitter in picomoles released in a 3-min collection period. See Knoll *et al.* (1996c) for methodology. Paired Student's *t*-test was used for statistical analysis. *$P<0.01$, **$P<0.001$.

3 min   ¤ electrical stimulation

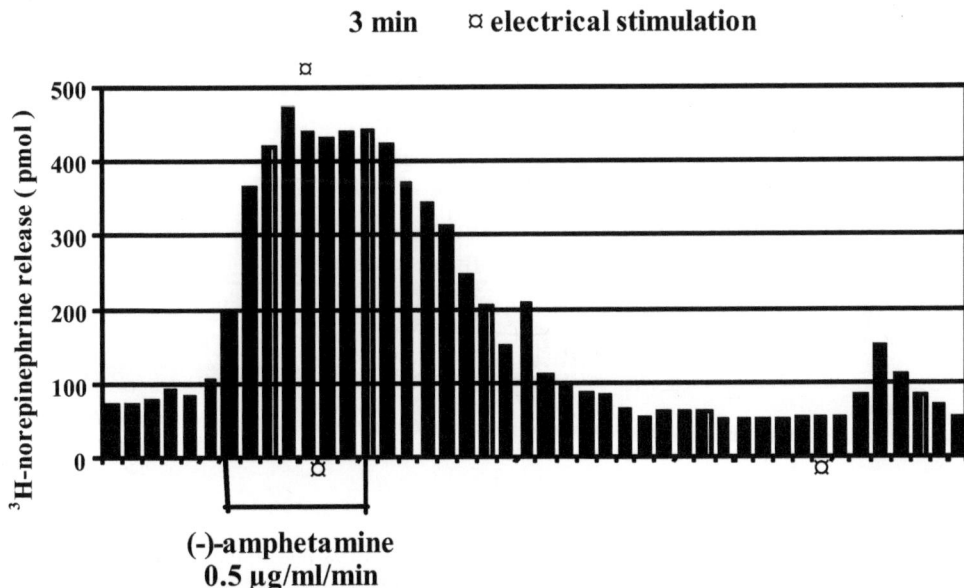

**(-)-amphetamine
0.5 µg/ml/min**

Figure 5: Demonstration that (-)-amphetamine, which in contrast to (-)-deprenyl preserved the norepinephrine-releasing property of PEA, their parent compound, is inducing a long lasting spontaneous release of ^{3}[H]-norepinephrine from an isolated rat brain stem. Electrical stimulation of the organ at the peak of the norepinephrine-releasing effect is ineffective thus the enhancer effect is undetectable.

□ 3 min   ¤ electrical stimulation

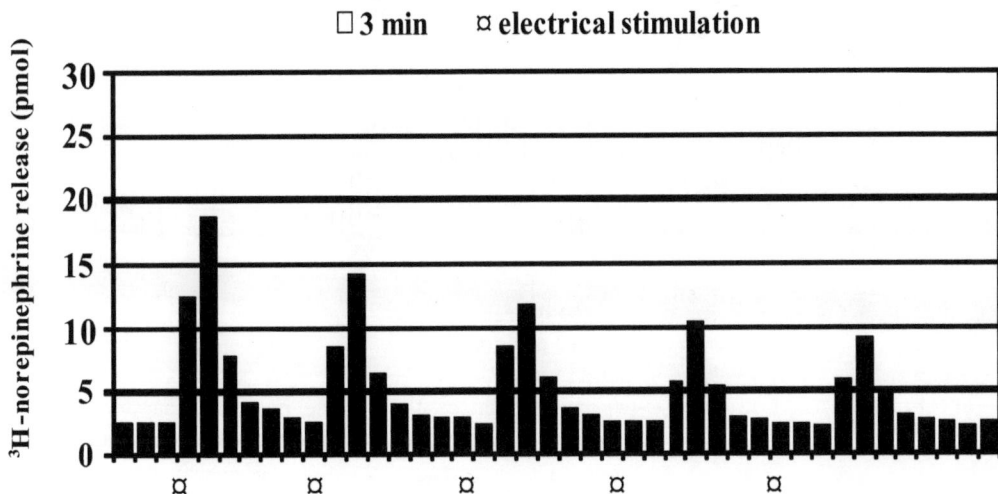

Figure 6: Release of ^{3}[H]-norepinephrine from an isolated rat brain stem to consecutive electrical stimulations. The figure shows that, due obviously to exhaustion, the amount of ^{3}[H]-norepinephrine released from the organ to electrical stimulation is, with the passing of time, on a gradual decline.

⊢3 min   ◻ electrical stimulation

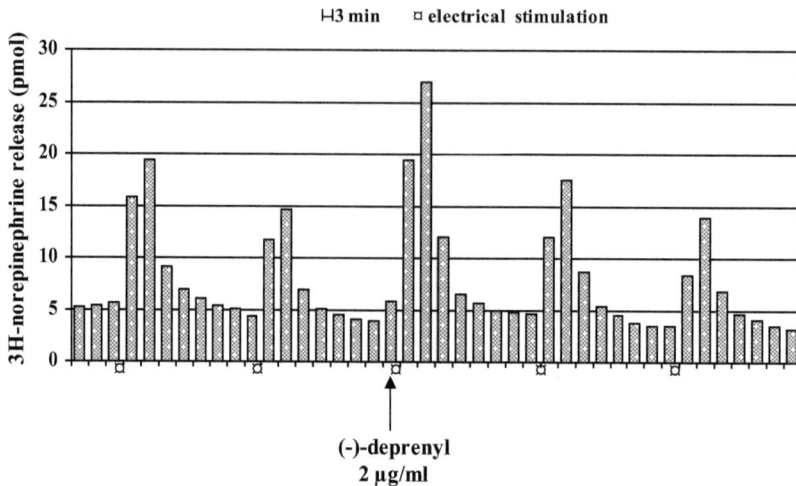

Figure 7: Demonstration that (-)-deprenyl, the unique PEA/(-)-methamphetamine-derivative, devoid of the catecholamine-releasing property of its parent compounds, allows to detect the CAE effect.

⊢ 3 min   ◻ electrical stimulation

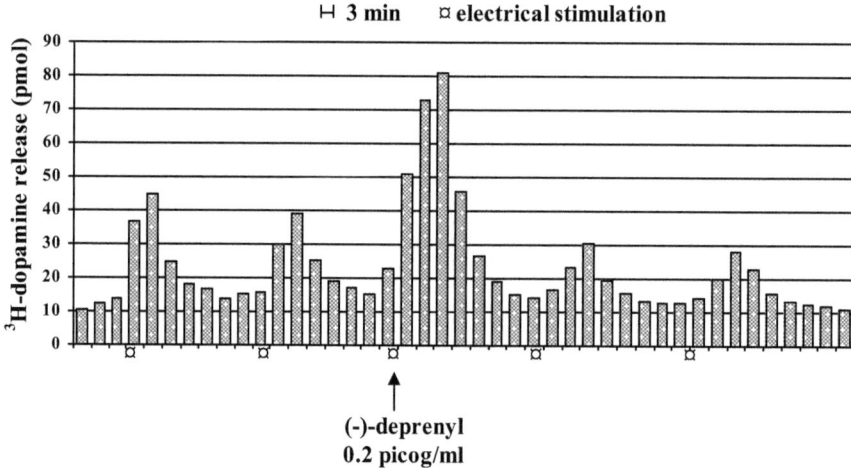

Figure 8: Demonstration that (-)-deprenyl enhances the release of ^{3}[H]-dopamine from the isolated rat brain stem to electrical stimulation in an extremely low concentration (0.2 picog/ml).

(-)-Deprenyl, enhances preferentially the activity of the catecholaminergic neurons in the brain stem. It selectively blocks the activity of MAO-B in the brain in a subcutaneous dose of 0.25 mg/kg. (-)-Deprenyl significantly enhances the impulse propagation mediated release of norepinephrine and dopamine from their neurons in the brain stem in a dose of 0.025 mg/kg (see for example Figs. **3** and **4** in Knoll 2005). This low dose of (-)-deprenyl leaves the physiological activity of B-type MAO practically unchanged.

The discovery that tryptamine is, like PEA, a natural enhancer substance (Knoll, 1994), initiated the structure-activity-relationship study resulting finally in the development of (-)-BPAP, a tryptamine-derived enhancer substance (Knoll *et al.*, 1999). Fig. **9** shows the chemical structure of (-)-BPAP.

(-)-BPAP enhances the release of dopamine from the substantia nigra of rats in a subcutaneous dose of 0.0001 mg/kg. In contrast to (-)-deprenyl it is a highly potent enhancer of the serotonergic neurons (see Figs. **8** and **9** in Knoll, 2005).

To date, (-)-BPAP is the most selective and potent experimental tool to investigate the enhancer regulation in the catecholaminergic and serotonergic neurons of the brain stem. The enhancer effect can be detected following the subcutaneous administration of low amounts of (-)-BPAP (see Table **2** in Knoll *et al.*, 1999,), as well as, following the addition of the substance into the organ bath of freshly isolated discrete brain areas (see Table **3** in Knoll *et al.*, 1999).

Enhancer substances stimulate the enhancer-sensitive neurons in the brain stem in a peculiar manner. Fig. **10** shows the characteristics of the enhancer effect of (-)-BPAP added to isolated locus coerulei of rats. The results show two bell-shaped concentration/effect curves. The one with a peak effect at 10^{-13}M concentration clearly demonstrates the existence of a highly complex, *specific* form of enhancer regulation in noradrenergic neurons. The second, with a peak effect at 10^{-6}M concentration, shows the operation of an obviously *nonspecific* form of the enhancer regulation in these neurons (see Knoll *et al.*, 2002, for details).

We found the same dose-effect relation regarding the specific enhancer effect of (-)-BPAP in *in vivo* experiments. We treated rats with saline or a single dose of 0.05, 0.0025, 0.0005, and 0.0001 mg/kg (-)-BPAP, respectively. 30 minutes after the subcutaneous injection, we quickly removed the locus coeruleus and measured, according to Knoll and Miklya (1995), the amount of norepinephrine released from the tissue within 20 minutes. In this experiment, the most effective dose of

(-)-BPAP, 0.0005 mg/kg, increased the release of norepinephrine from 4.7 ± 0.10 nM/g (control) to 15.4 ± 0.55 nM/g ($P<0.001$), but a 100-times higher dose of (-)-BPAP (0.05 mg/kg) did not change it (4.3 ± 0.25 nM/g) (Knoll *et al.*, 2002).

We experienced, in a number of studies on rats (Knoll *et al.*, 1955a,b,c, 1956, 1994; Knoll, 1956, 1957, 1988) the validity of the common concept that there is a great individual variation in sexual activity and learning performance in any random population of mammals of the same strain. For example, in our second longevity study (Knoll *et al.*, 1994) we selected from a population of sexually inexperienced 1600 Wistar-Logan rats the ones with the lowest sexual potency and found 94 rats which did not display in four consecutive weekly mating test any sign of sexual activity. We observed their copulatory activity in the presence of a female with high receptivity during 30 minutes and counted the copulatory patterns of the male (mounting, intromission and ejaculation). The "non-copulators" remained inactive until they died. On the other hand, we found 99 males which displayed at least one ejaculation in each of the four tests.

The discovery of the bell-shaped concentration/effect curve of the enhancer substance, in the low nanomolar concentration range, offers the first reasonable explanation for the great individual variation in behavioral performances. Since an *optimum* concentration of the enhancer substance was needed for the *optimum* performance, *I postulate that the substantial individual differences in behavioral performances are due to the peculiar dose-dependency of the endogenous enhancer substances.*

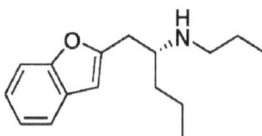

Systematic (IUPAC) name: (2*R*)-1-(1-benzofuran-2-yl)-*N*-propylpentane-2-amine

Figure 9: Chemical structure of (-)-BPAP.

This approach granted us a new perspective on the results of our two longitudinal studies performed on rats (first longevity study: Knoll, 1988; Knoll *et al.*, 1989; second longevity study; Knoll *et al.*, 1994).

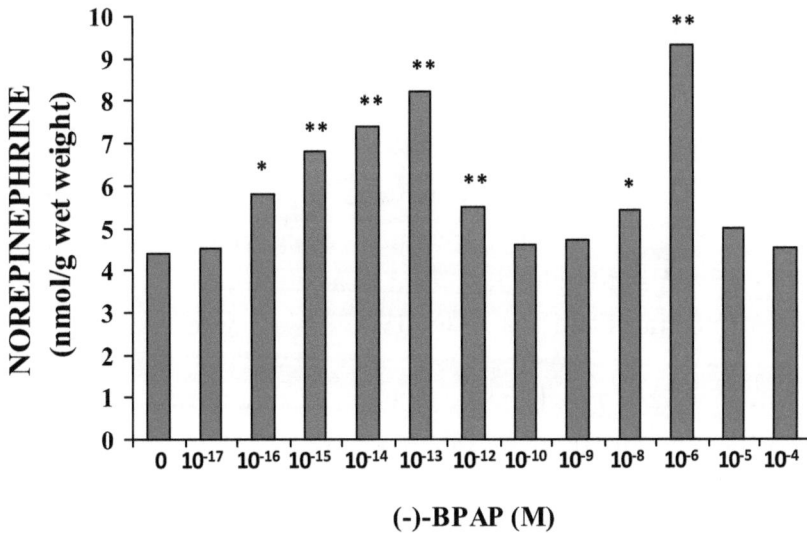

Figure 10: The bi-modal, bell-shaped concentration effect curve characteristic to the enhancer effect of (-)-BPAP on isolated locus coerulei of rats. (-)-BPAP was given to the organ bath of the quickly removed locus coerulei. Eight organs were used for the analysis of each concentration. The amount of norepinephrine released within 20 minutes from the tissue in the presence of different concentrations of (-)-BPAP was measured according to Knoll & Miklya (1995). Paired Student's *t*-test. *$P<0.01$, **$P<0.001$.

In the years when we performed our two longevity studies and worked with the robust Wistar-Logan rats, we observed that the males which completed the second year of their life did never display in the weekly mating test a single ejaculation. We experienced later that the Sprague-Dawley CFY or Wistar (Charles-River) rats too lost this ability at this age. Our studies clarified that the aging-related irresistible decay of the dopaminergic brain machinery is responsible for this change. Saline-treated CFY male rats reached the stage of unability to ejaculate at an average of 112 ± 9 weeks, their (-)-deprenyl-treated peers reached that stage at an average of 150 ± 12 weeks (Knoll, 1993a).

In our first longevity study we started to work with 132 sexually inexperienced 2-year old males and we tested their copulatory activity in four consecutive weekly mating tests during the 24th month of their life. According to their screening the rats were divided in three groups: 46 "non-copulators", 42 "mounting" rats and 44 "sluggish"rats (displaying mountings and intromissions). Thereafter we treated 66 rats with saline and 66 rats with 0.25 mg/kg (-)-deprenyl, three times a week, and observed their behavioral performances to the end of their life. We observed the rats until they died.

In the saline-treated group of the "non-copulators" died out first, the "mounting" rats lived longer, the longest living rats were in the "sluggish" group (see Table VI in Knoll 1988). (-)-Deprenyl treatment prolonged the life in each group significantly. The 66 salt-treated rats lived in average 147.05± 0.56 weeks, the 66 (-)-deprenyl-treated rats lived in average 197.98± 2.31 weeks.

The fact that the saline-treated "non-copulators" died out first and the finding that (-)-deprenyl, the special stimulant of the catecholaminergic brain stem neurons, keeps the rats on a higher activity level and prolongs their life, suggested that the catecholaminergic engine of the brain, which is of crucial importance in activating the cortex, is responsible for the lifespan-prolonging effect. Thus, the brain engine works in the 2-year old "non-copulator" males on a lower activity level than in the 2-year old "sluggish" males. This working hypothesis, based on the results of the first longevity study, determined the planning of the second longevity study. *We decided to start the experiment with younger rats, select from a huge population of Wistar-Logan rats the "non-copulators" and the sexually most active males, measure their sexual potency and learning ability until the end of their life, and treat the rats with saline and (-)-deprenyl, respectively.*

We started working with a random population of 28-week-old male rats and tested their sexual performance once a week. Rats that represented the two extremes in performance were selected for the study: the ones that did not display a single intromission during the four consecutive weekly-mating tests used for selection, and the ones which showed full scale sexual activity (mounting, intromission, ejaculation) in each of the four tests. Out of 1,600 sexually inexperienced 28-week-old Wistar-Logan male rats, that met a receptive female once a week during four consecutive weeks, 94 did not display a single intromission during the selection period and 99 displayed at least one ejaculation in each of the four tests. The former were taken for the lowest sexually performing (LP) rats, and the latter for the highest performing (HP) ones.

After selection we started to treat the 8-month-old rats subcutaneously with either 1 ml/kg 0.9% NaCl or with 0.25 mg/kg (-)-deprenyl, dissolved in 0.9% NaCl given in the same volume, three times a week, until the end of their life. Out of the 94 LP animals, 46 were treated with salt. Out of the 99 HP animals, 49 were treated with salt. The mating and learning performances of these salt-treated LP and HP rats were tested during a period of 108 weeks. Copulatory activity was tested once a week. The learning performance of the rats was tested in the shuttle box. The rats were trained once every three months for a period of five days, with 20 trials a day. In this longevity study we trained our rats in the shuttle box instead of the optimal training conditions (100 trial), only with 20 trials, to find more pronounced difference in the learning ability between high and low performing rats.

Fig. **11** demonstrates the highly significant difference in sexual and learning performances and in life span between LP and HP rats.

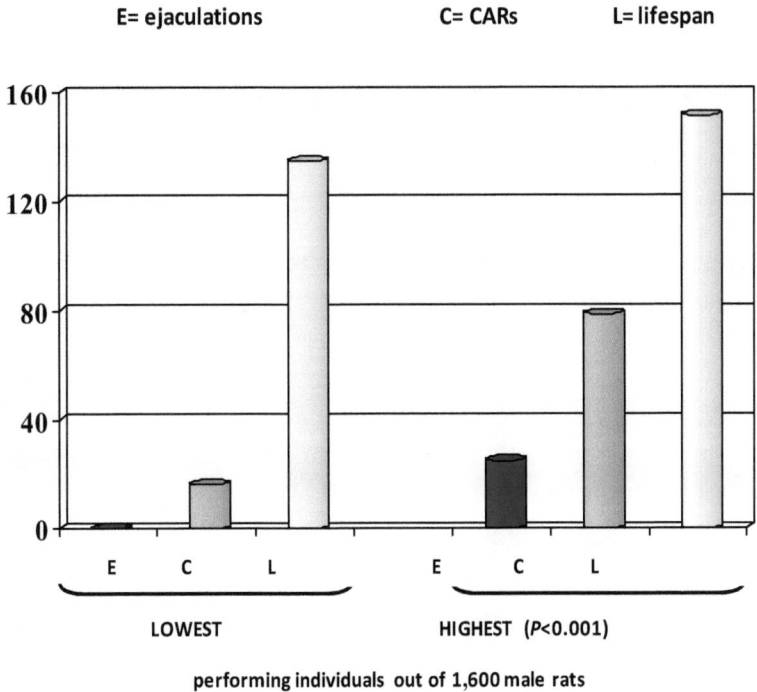

Figure 11: Illustration of the highly significant differences in sexual and learning performances and in lifespan between two groups of rats selected out of 1,600 28-week-old Wistar-Logan males, as the sexually lowest performing (LP) and highest performing (HP) individuals. See text for details.

The salt-treated LP rats (n=44) never displayed ejaculation during their lifetime, they were extremely dull in the shuttle box and lived 134.58±2.29 weeks. The salt-treated HP rats (n=49) displayed 14.04±0.56 ejaculations during the first 36-week testing period and due to aging they produced 2.47±0.23 ejaculations between the 73-108th week of testing. They lived 151.24±1.36 weeks, significantly (*P*<0.001) longer than their LP peers.

Maintenance on (-)-deprenyl enhanced the performance of both LP and HP rats and prolonged their lifespan significantly. The (-)-deprenyl-treated LP rats (n=48) became sexually active, their mating performance was substantially increased and lived 152.54±1.36 weeks, significantly longer than their salt-treated peers and as long as the salt-treated HP rats. The (-)-deprenyl-treated HP rats (n=50) were sexually much more active than their salt-treated peers. They displayed 30.04±0.85 ejaculations during the first 36-week testing period and 7.40±0.32 ejaculations between the 73-108th week of testing. Also their learning performance was substantially increased. They produced 113.98±3.23 CARs during the first 36-week-testing period and 81.68±2.14 CARs during the 73-108th week of testing. They lived 185.30±1.96 weeks, significantly more than their salt-treated peers and out of the 50 rats 17 lived longer than the estimated technical lifespan (TLS).

Considering the unique dose-related effect of an enhancer substance, we assume that out of the 1,600 rats, 99 HP rats produced their endogenous enhancer substances at the peak of the bell-shaped concentration/effect curve, while the 94 LP rats produced them at the least active part of the curve. The overwhelming majority of the population (1,407 rats) falls between these two extremes.

An analysis of the ability of rats to acquire the glass-cylinder-seeking drive is another example that convincingly illustrates the great individual differences in the behavioral performances of rat (see Sect. 1.3 and 4.2. in Knoll, 2005). We observed only in two rats out of 100 that the acquired glass-cylinder-seeking function operated lifelong with unchanged intensity. Presumably the specific endogenous enhancer substances in the cortical neurons responsible for the operation of the glass-cylinder-seeking drive were mobilized in these two rats in the optimum concentration. Thus regarding the measured function we may look upon these two rats as the most talented in the tested population.

There is a gleam of hope that better understanding of the enhancer regulation in the cortical neurons may finally allow to define on a molecular level the physiological mechanism responsible of "man of talent"/"genius". As analyzed and discussed in detail in my monograph (Knoll, 2005), since the natural endowments of the healthy human brain are identical, everybody is born with 100 billion neurons and 10^{11} bit capacity, everybody has necessarily brilliant abilities which remain unexplored, unutilized.

All in all, the discovery that PEA is a natural enhancer of the catecholaminergic and serotonergic neurons in the brain stem, and the fact that we successfully fabricated a much more potent and selective enhancer substance than (-)-deprenyl, is a heavy argument for the thesis that enhancer regulation operates in the catecholaminergic and serotonergic neurons in the brain and places at our disposal tools through which we can maintain the activity of enhancer-sensitive cells on higher activity level without changing their physiological milieu (see further analysis in Chapter 9).

As it will be discussed in Chapter 3 in detail, the enhancer regulation of the catecholaminergic and the serotonergic neurons in the brain starts working on a significantly higher activity level after weaning, and the intensified activity subsists until sexual maturity is reached; thereafter activity returns to the preweaning level. Developmental longevity is the phase between weaning and sexual maturity, the uphill period of life. Sexual hormones dampen the intensified enhancer regulation in the catecholaminergic and serotonergic neurons in the brain. Activity returns to the preweaning level and this is the transition from adolescence to adulthood. The postdevelopmental period, the downhill period of life begins, and lasts until natural death. During the postdevelopmental period, the enhancer regulation in the catecholaminergic brain machinery is on a slow continuous decline. The catecholaminergic neurons play a key role in the efficiency of learning performances, drive motivated behavior, *etc.* The continuous decline of their activity with the passing of time plays a crucial role in the behavioral consequences of brain aging.

Since with the daily preventive administration of a synthetic enhancer substance from sexual maturity until death we can maintain the activity of the catecholaminergic and serotonergic neurons on a higher activity level, we have a chance to slow safely the aging-related decay of physical and mental welfare.

Send Orders of Reprints at reprints@benthamscience.org

CHAPTER 3

The Catecholaminergic Control of the Uphill and Downhill Period of Life

There are good reasons to assume that it is the physiological role of the catecholaminergic neurons to keep the higher brain centers in a continuously active state, the intensity of which is dynamically changed within broad limits according to need. Such regulation is the condition *sine qua non* for the integrative work of the CNS. The operation of the catecholaminergic system is comparable to an engine which is ignited once for an entire lifetime, as signaled by the appearance of the EEG, in an early phase of development.

Due to aging, the maximum level of activation of the CNS, *via* the catecholaminergic system, decreases progressively with the passing of time. The blackout ("natural death") of the integrative work of the CNS, signaled by the disappearance of the EEG, occurs when the catecholaminergic system's ability to activate the higher brain centers sinks below a critical threshold and an emergency incident transpires, when a high level of activation is needed to survive and the CNS can no longer be activated to the required extent. This would explain why a common infection, a broken leg, or any other challenge easily surmountable given catecholaminergic machinery at full capacity may cause death in old age.

The essence of this hypothesis is depicted in Fig. **12**. According to this scheme, the life of a mammalian organism can be divided, from a functional point of view, into six stages, each beginning with a qualitative change of crucial importance. The first stage starts with the fertilization of the ovum and lasts until the catecholaminergic system properly activates the higher levels of the brain, which then take the lead and integrate the different parts of the organism into a highly sophisticated entity. We may deem the first stage of development of the mammalian organism as being completed when the catecholaminergic engine of the brain is put into gear once and for all. This is the intrauterine birth of the unique individual. The appearance of the EEG signals the transition from the first into the second stage of development.

Cells need oxygen, water, and food for life. These are first supplied, *via* the placenta, by the mother. The subsequent, highly complicated evolving program is devoted to ensuring independence from the mother.

The second stage of development ends with the passage of the fetus from the uterus to the outside world. From a functional point of view birth means the transition from fetal to postnatal circulation, with the newborn infant now supplying itself with oxygen.

The third stage lasts from birth until weaning and serves to develop the skills needed for the maintenance of integrity and for the infant to supply itself with water and food.

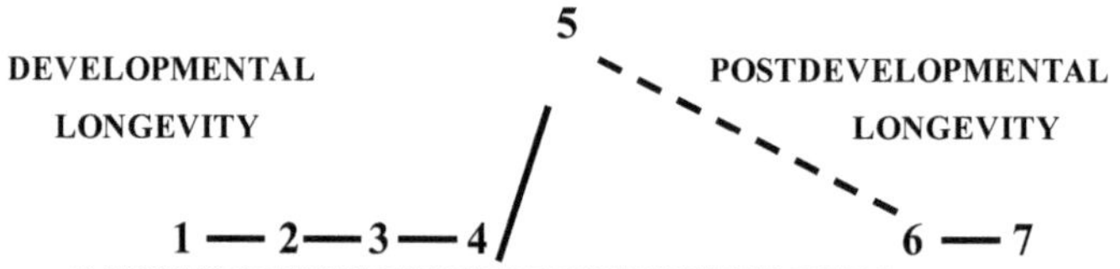

```
                                5
      DEVELOPMENTAL                 POSTDEVELOPMENTAL
        LONGEVITY                       LONGEVITY

          1 — 2 — 3 — 4/                    6 — 7
        1) FUSION OF THE SPERMATOZOON WITH THE OVUM
        2) THE INTEGRATIVE WORK OF THE CNS SETS IN.
           APPEARENCE OF EEG
        3) BIRTH OF THE FOETUS
        4) WEANING
        5) SEXUAL MATURITY IS REACHED
        6) THE INTEGRATIVE WORK OF THE CNS BLACKS OUT.
           DISAPPEARANCE OF EEG. 'NATURAL DEATH'
        7) DEATH OF THE LAST CELL
```

Figure 12: Conception about essential changes during the lifetime of mammals.

The fourth stage lasts from weaning until the goal of goals in nature, full scale sexual maturity is reached. This is the most delightful phase of life, the glorious uphill journey. The individual progressively takes possession, on a mature level, of all abilities crucial for survival and maintenance of the species. It learns to avoid dangerous situations, masters the techniques for obtaining its food, develops procreative powers for sexual reproduction and copulates. This is, at the same time, the climax of developmental longevity.

The sexually fully mature individual fulfils its duty. Thus, to maintain the precisely balanced natural equilibrium among living organisms, the biologically "useless" individual has to be eliminated. According to the inborn program, the fifth, postdevelopmental stage of life (aging) begins.

The essence of the fifth stage is progressive decay of the efficiency of the catecholaminergic system during the postdevelopmental lifespan until at some point, in an emergency situation, the integration of the parts in a highly sophisticated entity can no longer be maintained and "natural death", signaled by the disappearance of the EEG signal, sets in.

As parts of the organism remain alive, the sixth and last stage of life is the successive dying off of the different groups of cells.

The hypothesis outlined suggests that quality and duration of life rests upon the inborn efficiency of the catecholaminergic brain machinery, *i.e.*, a higher performing, longer-living individual has a more active, more slowly deteriorating catecholaminergic system than its low performing, shorter-living peer. To simplify this concept, we may say, that a better brain engine allows for a better performance and a longer lifespan. *The concept clearly predicts that, as the activity of the catecholaminergic system can be improved at any time during life, it must essentially be feasible to develop a technique for transforming a lower-performing, shorter-living individual, to a better-performing, longer-living one. It therefore follows that a shift of the duration of life beyond the technical lifespan (TLS), with a yet unpredictable upper limit, must be possible in all mammals, including the human species.* The results of the longevity study (Knoll *et al.*, 1994), reviewed in detail in Chapter 2, are in harmony with this concept.

What is the cause of the transition from developmental to postdevelopmental longevity? This is the main question to be answered.

To answer this question we need to consider a phenomenon of which we first took notice in the course of our behavioral studies on rats performed in the 1950s. We observed that hunger drive induced orienting-searching reflex activity was significantly more pronounced in young rats than in their elder peers (Knoll, 1957). We repeatedly corroborated this observation later and described it for the last time in 1995 (Knoll & Miklya, 1995.)

Catecholaminergic neurons have a powerful activating effect on the brain. We measured hunger-induced orienting-searching reflex activity in rats and found that animals in the late developmental phase of life (2 months of age) were much more active than those in the early postdevelopmental phase (4 months of age), which points to the enhanced catecholaminergic activity during the developmental phase.

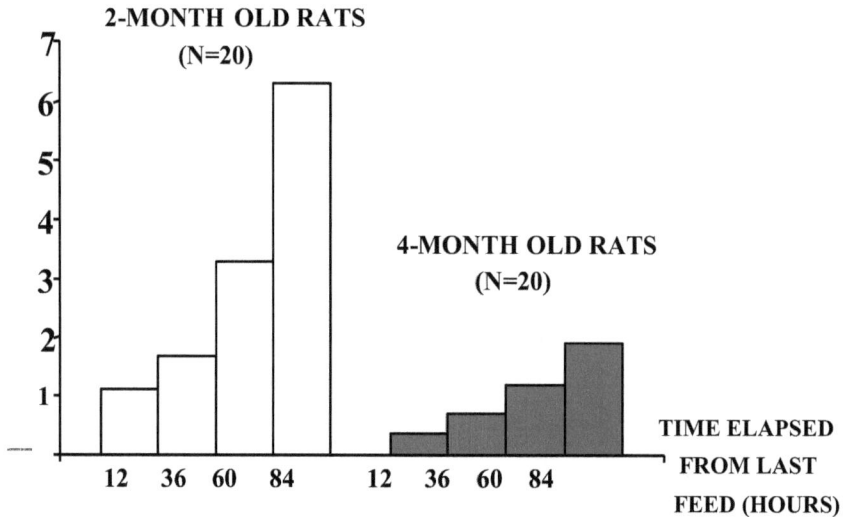

Figure 13: Intensity of orienting-searching reflex activity of hungry rats in surroundings quite new to them as a function of time elapsed from last feed. Activity was measured and expressed in units from 0 to 10. See Knoll & Miklya (1995) for methodology and other details.

Fig. **13** shows that if we measure the intensity of orienting-searching reflex activity of hungry rats in a new surrounding as a function of time elapsed from the last feed, we observe the striking difference in activity between rats being in their uphill period of life (2-month-old animals) and 4-month-old rats being already in their early postdevelopmental phase of life. We also observed the awakening of sexual drive, maturation of spermatozoa and the development of the penis in male CFY rats. From the strain we used in this experiment, it was exceptional to find copulatory drive manifesting in males younger than six weeks. Although the appearance of copulatory patterns usually precedes maturation of spermatozoa and full development of the penis, the overwhelming majority of the males reached full-scale sexual activity by the completion of their 2nd month of life.

In the rat, the interval from weaning (3rd week of life) until the end of the 2nd month of age is a decisive period for the development of the individual. During this period the animal acquires abilities crucial for survival and maintenance of the species.

Based on the observation that the 2-month-old hungry rats are significantly more active than their 4-month-old peers, we checked their dopaminergic, noradrenergic and serotonergic activities in the brain before weaning (in 2-week-old rats), during the crucial developmental phase, from weaning to sexual maturity (in 4- and 8-week-old rats) and in the early postdevelopmental phase of life (in 16- and 32-week-old rats). As an indicator of the basic activity of catecholaminergic and serotonergic neurons in the brain, we measured the release of dopamine from striatum, substantia nigra and tuberculum olfactorium, of norepinephrine from the locus coeruleus, and of serotonin from the raphe, in male and female rats (Knoll & Miklya, 1995).

We found that from weaning until the 2nd month of life the striatal dopaminergic system of the rats was significantly more active than either before or after that period. Fig. **14** demonstrates a dramatic increase in the release of dopamine from the striatum and tuberculum olfactorium after weaning (4th week) and the return of the release of dopamine to the preweaning leve (2nd week) in sexually mature rats (32nd week). This explains why, as demonstrated in Fig. **13**, food-deprived rats in their developmental phase of life were significantly more mobile in an open field than their peers already in their early postdevelopmental phase of life. Our finding regarding the age-related changes in the dopaminergic tone in the rat brain was confirmed on Long Evans Cinnamon rats (Samuele *et al.*, 2005, Table **4**).

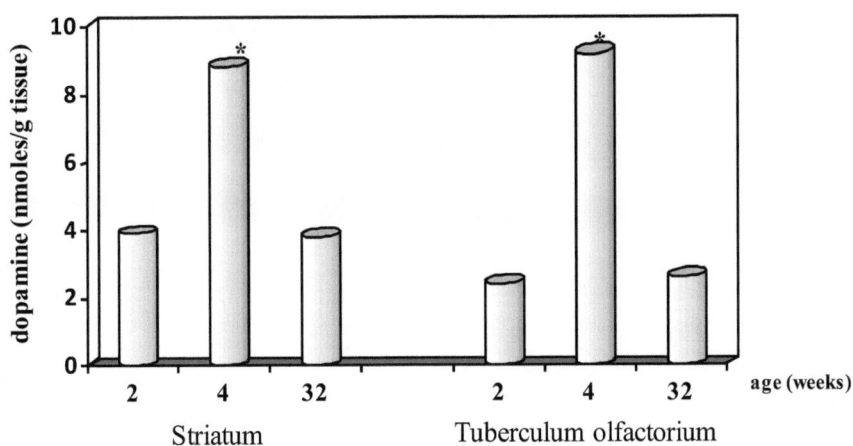

Figure 14: Release of dopamine from the striatum and tuberculum olfactorium, respectively, of male rats belonging to different age cohorts. N=12; * $P<0.001$. For details see Knoll & Miklya (1995).

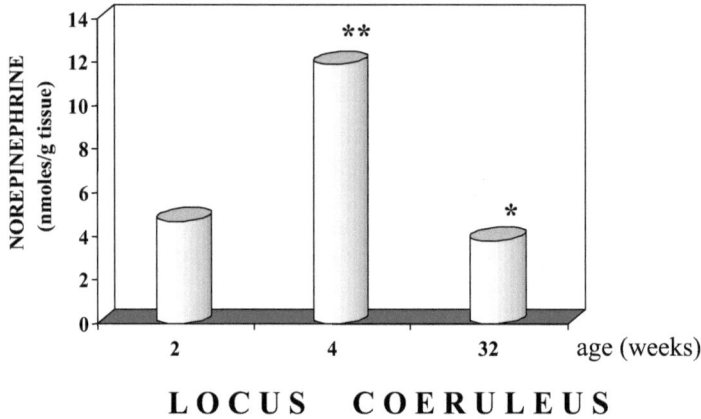

Figure 15: Release of norepinephrine from the locus coeruleus of male rats belonging to different age cohorts. N=12; * *P<0.01,* **P <0.001. For details see Knoll & Miklya (1995).

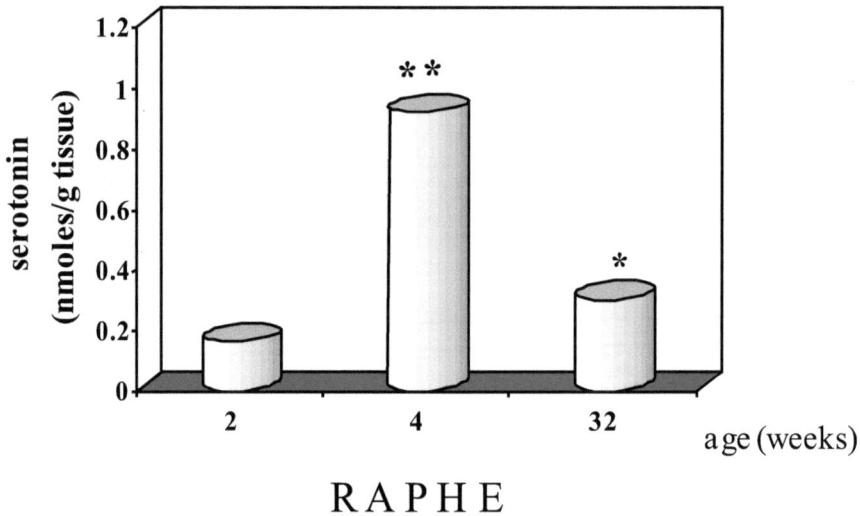

Figure 16: Release of serotonin from the raphe of male rats belonging to different age cohorts. N=12; * *P<0.01* **P <0.001. For details see Knoll & Miklya (1995).

The release of norepinephrine from the locus coeruleus (Fig. **15**) and the release of serotonin from the raphe (Fig. **16**) show the same dramatic increase after weaning and the return to the preweaning level in sexually mature rats as dopamine (for details see Knoll & Miklya, 1995).

All in all, we found that enhancer regulation starts working on a higher activity level after weaning, and this state of enhanced activity continues in existence until the completion of full scale sexual development, with a rapid rate of decay thereafter. It is obvious that as soon as sexual maturity was reached the catecholaminergic tone changes from a "hyperactive" to an "economy" state, signaling the transition from a developmental to a postdevelopmental (aging) phase of life. We may also conclude that enhanced enhancer regulation between weaning and sexual maturity is responsible for the exuberant physical strength and mental vigor of mammals in their uphill period of life.

Since we measured in both male and female rats a significantly more pronounced enhancer regulation in the dopaminergic, noradrenergic and serotonergic neurons from the discontinuation of breast feeding (end of the 3rd week of age) until the appearance of sexual hormones (end of the 2nd month of life), it was reasonable to deduce that sexual hormones play the key role in terminating the developmental phase of life (Knoll *et al.*, 2000).

The regulation of sexual hormones starts working in the rat with full capacity only at the end of the 2nd month of age. This rapid decrease in norepinephrine, dopamine and serotonin from selected discrete brain regions appeared synchronously with the completion of sexual maturity. Thus, it was reasonable to assume that sexual hormones dampen the enhancer regulation in the catecholaminergic and serotonergic brain stem neurons, and this is the mechanism which terminates developmental longevity as well.

In order to qualify these observations we castrated three-week-old male and female rats and measured the release of catecholamines and serotonin from selected discrete brain regions at the end of the third month of their life. We found that in male rats the amount of catecholamines and serotonin released from the neurons was significantly higher in castrated than in untreated or sham operated rats, signaling that sex hormones inhibit enhancer regulation in the brain (Table **3**).

To further analyze this effect of sex hormones, we treated male and female rats subcutaneously with oil (0.1 ml/rat), testosterone (0.1 mg/rat), estrone (0.01 mg/rat) and progesterone (0.5 mg/rat), respectively, and measured their effect on the enhancer regulation. Twenty-four hours after a single injection with the hormones, the release of norepinephrine, dopamine and serotonin was significantly inhibited in the testosterone-, or estrone-treated rats (Table **4**), but remained unchanged after progesteron treatment (Table **5**). In rats treated with a single hormone injection, testosterone in the male and estrone in the female were the significantly more effective inhibitors. Remarkably, the reverse order of potency was found in rats treated with daily hormone injections for 7 or 14 days (Tables **6** and **7**). After a two-week treatment with the hormones, estrone was found in the male and testosterone in the female as the significantly more potent inhibitors of the enhancer regulation.

The data prove that sex hormones terminate the hyperactive phase of life by dampening enhancer regulation in the catecholaminergic and serotonergic neurons. They bring about the transition from the developmental phase of life to postdevelopmental longevity, from adolescence to adulthood. This change is in the meantime also the beginning of the slow, continuous decay of the enhancer regulation in catecholaminergic and serotonergic neurons in the brain stem. As a consequence of it, the fixation of inextinguishable conditioned reflexes (ICRs) and the acquisition of drives are subject of an irresistible, slowly progressing, age-related decline until death.

Although the individual variation in decline of behavioral performances with passing time is substantial, the process hits every brain. Both the decay in brain performances as well as the potential for the manifestation of aging-related neurodegenerative diseases (Parkinson's, Alzheimer's) increase with the physiologically irrepressible aging of the brain. It is obvious that only the development of a safe and efficient preventive pharmacological intervention, starting immediately after the completion of sexual maturity, can significantly slow brain aging.

Hayflick mentioned in his "Theories of biological aging" that "It is possible that only by increasing lifespan, or maximum age of death, of members of a species, will important insight be made into the aging process" (Hayflick, 1985). Since in our two longevity studies, performed with (-)-deprenyl on the robust Wistar-Logan rats, some lived beyond the estimated maximum age of death, better understanding of the enhancer regulation in the brain might be helpful in the future to find efficient means to prolong human life beyond the TLS. This would be a groundbreaking example of man's endeavor to outwit Nature by understanding the laws of its operation.

Table 3: The release of catecholamines and serotonin from selected discrete brain regions isolated from the brain of 3-month-old male and female rats, untreated, sham operated or castrated at the age of 3-weeks.

MALES	Amount of Biogenic Amine (Nmoles/g Tissue) Released from the Tissue within 20 Min				
	Dopamine			Norepinephrine	Serotonin
	Striatum	Substantia nigra	Tuberculum olfactorium	Locus coeruleus	Raphe
Untreated	3.4±0.008	4.8±0.17	3.5±0.15	3.9±0.12	0.334±0.01
Sham operated	3.3±0.11	5.2±0.34	3.5±0.16	3.9±0.09	0.329±0.02
Castrated	4.4±0.17**	7.4±0.21**	4.7±0.12**	5.5±0.22**	0.921±0.02**
FEMALES					
Untreated	3.0±0.14	4.5±0.14	2.9±0.05	3.1±0.07	0.337±0.01
Sham operated	2.9±0.13	4.3±0.17	2.8±0.18	3.0±0.05	0.339±0.01
Castrated	4.6±0.29**	8.3±0.18**	3.7±0.06**	4.40±0.05**	0.491±0.03*

Paired Student's t-test. N=16.

$*P<0.02$; $**P<0.001$

Table 4: The release of catecholamines and serotonin from selected discrete brain regions isolated from the brain of 4-week-old male and female rats 24 hours after a single subcutaneous injection with oil (0.1 ml/rat), testosterone proprionate (0.1 mg/rat) and estrone (0.01 mg/rat), respectively

MALES	Amount of Biogenic Amine (Nmoles/g Tissue) Released from the Tissue Within 20 Min				
	Dopamine			Norepinephrine	Serotonin
	Striatum	Substantia Nigra	Tuberculum Olfactorium	Locus Coeruleus	Raphe
Vehicle (A)	6.6±0.23	11.8±0.23	6.8±0.21	9.6±0.19	1.178±0.14
Testosterone (B)	4.7±0.19	10.8±0.34	4.8±0.13	3.4±0.21	0.581±0.11
Estrone (C)	5.8±0.21	11.6±0.26	5.8±0.20	4.2±0.35	0.918±0.04
	A:B ****	A:B *	A:B ****	A:B ****	A:B **
	A:C *	A:C ⁻	A:C ***	A:C ****	A:C ⁻
	B:C **	B:C ⁻	B:C ***	B:C ⁻	B:C *
FEMALES					
Vehicle (A)	7.7±0.27	11.8±0.26	7.9±0.17	9.0±0.26	1.120±0.07
Testosterone (B)	6.8±0.45	11.4±0.21	7.1±0.35	4.7±0.37	0.815±0.09
Estrone (C)	5.5±0.16	11.2±0.39	6.3±0.39	3.7±0.32	0.377±0.11
	A:B ⁻	A:B ⁻	A:B ⁻	A:B ****	A:B *
	A:C ****	A:C ⁻	A:C ***	A:C ****	A:C ***
	B:C ***	B:C ⁻	B:C ⁻	B:C ⁻	B:C *

Paired Student's t-test. N=16.

$⁻P>0.05$; $*P<0.05$; $**P<0.02$; $*** P<0.01$; $**** P<0.001$.

Table 5: The release of catecholamines and serotonin from selected discrete brain regions isolated from the brain of 4-week-old male and female rats, 24 hours after a single subcutaneous injection with oil (0.1 ml/rat) and progesterone (0.5 mg/rat), respectively

MALES	Amount of Biogenic Amine (Nmoles/g Tissue) Released from the Tissue Within 20 Min				
	Dopamine			Norepinephrine	Serotonin
	Striatum	Substantia Nigra	Tuberculum Olfactorium	Locus Coeruleus	Raphe
Vehicle	5.9±0.27	10.4±0.22	6.2±0.31	9.9±0.70	1.071±0.11
Progesterone	5.7±0.20	10.6±0.33	5.9±0.08	10.0±0.05	1.026±0.07
	P>0.05	*P*>0.05	*P*>0.05	*P*>0.05	*P*>0.05
FEMALES					
Vehicle	5.8±0.13	10.5±0.29	6.4±0.21	10.8±0.10	1.080±0.02
Progesterone	5.8±0.15	10.1±0.30	6.2±0.22	10.4±0.80	1.470±0.03
	P>0.05	*P*>0.05	*P*>0.05	*P*>0.05	*P*>0.05

Paired Student's t-test. N=16.

Table 6: The release of catecholamines and serotonin from selected discrete brain regions isolated from the brain of male and female rats injected once daily for 7 days subcutaneously with oil (0.1 ml/rat), testosterone proprionate (0.1 mg/rat) and estrone (0.01 mg/rat), respectively

MALES	Amount of Biogenic Amine (Nmoles/g Tissue) Released from the Tissue Within 20 Min				
	Dopamine			Norepinephrine	Serotonin
	Striatum	Substantia Nigra	Tuberculum Olfactorium	Locus Coeruleus	Raphe
Vehicle (A)	6.2±0.24	11.9±0.37	7.1±0.18	9.5±0.20	0.914±0.04
Testosterone (B)	5.0±0.17	11.8±0.10	5.1±0.13	5.8±0.17	0.281±0.01
Estrone (C)	4.9±0.31	11.7±0.24	4.7±0.17	4.3±0.10	0.459±0.02
	A:B ***	A:B ⁻	A:B ****	A:B **	A:B ***
	A:C *	A:C ⁻	A:C ****	A:C ***	A:C ***
	B:C ⁻	B:C ⁻	B:C ⁻	B:C ⁻	B:C **
FEMALES					
Vehicle (A)	6.6±0.22	12.0±0.20	6.5±0.25	9.3±0.30	0.944±0.04
Testosterone (B)	3.4±0.13	10.9±0.23	4.6±0.26	5.2±0.05	0.236±0.02
Estrone (C)	5.4±0.11	10.3±0.11	5.9±0.18	5.0±0.05	0.520±0.01
	A:B ****	A:B ***	A:B ***	A:B ***	A:B ***
	A:C ***	A:C ****	A:C ⁻	A:C ***	A:C ***
	B:C ****	B:C ⁻	B:C ***	B:C ⁻	B:C ***

Treatment started on 3-week-old rats. Brain samples were isolated 24 hours after the last injection.

Paired Student's t-test. N=16.

⁻*P*>0.05; **P*<0.05; ***P*<0.02; *** *P*<0.01; **** *P*<0.001

Table 7: The release of catecholamines and serotonin from selected discrete brain regions isolated from the brain of male and female rats injected once daily for 14 days subcutaneously with oil (0.1 ml/rat), testosterone proprionate (0.1 mg/rat) and estrone (0.01 mg/rat), respectively

MALES	Amount of Biogenic Amine (Nmoles/g Tissue) Released from the Tissue Within 20 Min				
	Dopamine			Norepinephrine	Serotonin
	Striatum	Substantia nigra	Tuberculum olfactorium	Locus coeruleus	Raphe
Vehicle (A)	5.8±0.24	14.3±0.30	7.6±0.13	6.5±0.40	1.090±0.01
Testosterone (B)	6.4±0.28	13.0±0.19	5.8±0.24	5.6±0.10	0.415±0.01
Estrone (C)	4.6±0.21	9.8±0.27	5.6±0.21	2.0±0.10	0.213±0.02
	A:B ¯	A:B ***	A:B ****	A:B ¯	A:B ***
	A:C **	A:C ***	A:C ****	A:C ***	A:C ***
	B:C ***	B:C ****	B:C ¯	B:C ***	B:C **
FEMALES					
Vehicle (A)	5.1±0.06	11.7±0.13	6.2±0.15	6.7±0.25	1.007±0.01
Testosterone (B)	4.4±0.18	10.8±0.36	4.5±0.15	3.8±0.15	0.218±0.02
Estrone (C)	5.7±0.23	10.2±0.34	5.6±0.20	6.5±0.30	0.607±0.01
	A:B ***	A:B ¯	A:B ****	A:B ***	A:B ****
	A:C ¯	A:C ***	A:C *	A:C ¯	A:C ****
	B:C ***	B:C ¯	B:C ***	B:C **	B:C ***

Treatment started on 3-week-old rats. Brain samples were isolated 24 hours after the last injection.

Paired Student's t-test. N=16.

¯$P>0.05$; *$P<0.05$; **$P<0.02$; *** $P<0.01$; **** $P<0.001$

CHAPTER 4

The Antioxidant and Neuroprotective Effect of (-)-Deprenyl and their Relation to the Enhancer Effect

As discussed earlier the catecholaminergic and serotonergic neurons are excellent models to study the enhancer regulation. (-)-Deprenyl, the PEA-derived enhancer substance, which lost the catecholamine-releasing property of its parent compounds, PEA and (-)-methaphetamine (see Figs. **5, 6, 7**), was the specific experimental tool which allowed to realize the operation of the enhancer regulation in the catecholaminergic brain stem neurons. The discovery that tryptamine is like PEA a natural enhancer substance, and the development of (-)-BPAP, a much more potent enhancer substance than (-)-deprenyl, which in contrast to (-)-deprenyl is a highly potent enhancer of the serotonergic neurons as well, was final proof that the enhancer regulation operates in the catecholaminergic and serotonergic neurons in the brain.

The discovery of the enhancer regulation in these neurons is, however, obviously just the peak of an iceberg. We do not know how many natural enhancer-sensitive cellular mechanisms exist in mammalian organisms and which their natural regulators are. Our finding that PEA and tryptamine are endogenous enhancers and the development of their synthetic analogues, (-)-deprenyl and (-)-BPAP, are just the first examples that call our attention to the existence of previously unknown enhancer regulations in mammalian organisms.

Up to the present (-)-deprenyl is the only synthetic enhancer substance the effects of which have already been described in thousand of papers. Since (-)-deprenyl was the first selective inhibitor of MAO-B, the drug is still handled as the classic inhibitor of B-type MAO. In the brain of rats (-)-deprenyl blocks MAO-B in a dose of 0.25 mg/kg and exerts its specific enhancer effect on the catecholaminergic neurons in a dose of 0.001 mg/kg. Nevertheless, the CAE effect of (-)-deprenyl is so far left out of consideration.

Although it is obviously unreasonable to use higher than 0.25 mg/kg doses of (-)-deprenyl in animal experiments, there are still published studies in which

(-)-deprenyl is used in 1-10 mg/kg doses. This practice of raised levels of (-)-deprenyl exerts dozens of unwanted effects and leads to statements that (-)-deprenyl has amphetamine-like effects, is a releaser of catecholamines from their intraneuronal pools, blocks the reuptake of dopamine, *etc.* (-)-Deprenyl may block even catecholaminergic receptors in such high doses as 10 mg/kg. The optimal dose of (-)-deprenyl, which blocks already efficiently MAO-B activity selectively in the brain (0.25 mg/kg), is free of significant unwanted effects. The enhancer dose range, from 0.001 to 0.1 mg/kg, is devoid of noteworthy side effects. (-)-Deprenyl is a drug with an unusually broad safety margin. In animal experiment (-)-deprenyl exerts its specific enhancer effect in a dose as low as 0.001 mg/kg and even repeated daily doses of 10 mg/kg are exceptionally well tolerated.

Up to the present, hundreds of papers describe the protecting effect of (-)-deprenyl against neurotoxic agents, such as 6-hydroxydopamine (6-OHDA), 1-methyl-4-phenyl-1,2,3,6 tetrahydropyridine (MPTP), N-(2-chloroethyl)-N-ethyl-2-bromobenzylamine (DSP-4), and methyl-beta-acetoxyethyl-2-chloroethylamine (AF64-A).

It was first shown in the late 1970s that (-)-deprenyl-treatment protects the dopaminergic neurons from the toxic effect of the specific dopaminergic neurotoxin, 6-OHDA (Knoll, 1978; Harsing *et al.*, 1979, Knoll, 1987). The activity of the cholinergic interneurons in the caudate nucleus is continuously inhibited by dopamine, released in the striatum. This is the main physiological effect of striatal dopamine. In PD, due to the dopamine-deficiency-induced gradually declining inhibition of the cholinergic interneurons, higher amounts of acetylcholine (ACh) are liberated. Levodopa-treatment (dopamine supplementation) in PD restores the toppled physiological equilibrium. This chain of events can be followed in experiments with striatal slices taken from the brain stem of rats treated with 6-OHDA (see Table 6 in Knoll, 1987). The amount of ouabain-induced release of ACh from striatal slices dissected from untreated rats was found to be 366.7±57.3 pmole/g/min and the addition of dopamine (2.6 x 10^{-4} mole/L) increased the amount to 591.0±52.5 pmole/g/min, showing that dopamine stimulated the presynaptic dopamine "autoreceptors". In striatal slices taken from rats pretreated with 6-OHDA, the ouabain-induced release of ACh increased to 706.0±60.0 pmole/g/min, similarly to the situation in PD, where loss of the nigrostriatal dopaminergic neurons leads to an uninhibited release of ACh in the striatum. The addition of dopamine inhibited to 372.9±93.8 pmole/g/min the ouabain-induced release of ACh, thus acted in the model like levodopa acts in PD.

(-)-Deprenyl-treatment protected completely the striatum from the toxic effect of 6-OHDA. The subcutaneous injection of 0.25 mg/kg of (-)-deprenyl for 3 weeks and the administration of 6-OHDA for 24 hours after the last injection of (-)-deprenyl did not change the ouabain-induced release of ACh. It was the final conclusion of this paper that (-)-deprenyl protects the striatum from the toxic effects of 6-OHDA *via* the blockade of B-type MAO, the inhibition of the uptake of 6-OHDA into the neuron, the facilitation of scavenger function, and the improvement of the removal of the neurotoxic free radicals (Knoll, 1987, p.57). It was this finding which catalyzed the discovery that (-)-deprenyl is significantly enhancing the activity of superoxide dismutase (SOD) in the striatum of both male and female rats (Knoll, 1988).

All of these findings were thereafter confirmed in dozens of papers. It is now common knowledge that (-)-deprenyl protects dopaminergic neurons from the toxic effect of 6-OHDA and facilitates scavenger function in the dopaminergic neurons (for review see Miklya, 2011).

As it is well known today, it was discovered accidentally that drug addicts in California developed PD after self-administration of a "synthetic heroin" which was contaminated with MPTP. Langston *et al.,* first described that a chemist working with MPTP developed PD and demonstrated that pargyline, a semiselective inhibitor of B-type MAO, prevents MPTP-induced parkinsonism in primates (Langston & Ballard, 1983; Langston *et al.*, 1983, 1984). Markey *et al.,* suggested that intraneuronal generation of a pyridinium-metabolite may cause drug-induced parkinsonism (Markey *et al.*, 1984). It was soon demonstrated in a series of detailed studies that MPTP is oxidized by B-type of MAO first to 1-methyl-4-phenyl-2,3 dihydropyridinium ion ($MPDP^+$) and finally to methyl-phenyl-tetrahydro-pyridinium ion (MPP^+), which generates free radicals and causes parkinsonism in human beings. MPP^+ is selectively accumulated in mitochondria in the dopaminergic nerve terminals and acts like 6-OHDA. (-)-Deprenyl, as a selective inhibitor of B-type MAO, protects of course the dopaminergic neurons from the toxic effect of MPTP. This was first published in 1984 by Melvin Yahr's group in monkeys (Cohen *et al.*, 1984), in 1985 by Heikkila's group in mice (Heikkila *et al.*, 1985) and was thereafter confirmed many times.

It is obvious that the inhibition of MAO-B plays the key role in the protective effect of (-)-deprenyl against the neurotoxic effect of MPTP. Nevertheless, (-)-deprenyl enhances the production of neurotrophins [nerve growth factor (NGF), brain-derived neurotrophic factor (BDNF), glial-cell-line-derived neurotrophic factor (GDNF)] in glial cells – all of which are natural protective agents of the neurons. This glial effect of (-)-deprenyl is due to its enhancer effect. (-)-BPAP, the specific enhancer substance, is highly potent in increasing the production of neurotrophins in glial cells (Ohta *et al.*, 2002; Shimazu *et al.*, 2003). Thus, even in this case, the enhancer effect might be an additional factor in the effectiveness of (-)-deprenyl against MPTP toxicity.

Further studies revealed that (-)-deprenyl protects different neurons against a variety of neurotoxic agents: dopaminergic neurons against beta-carbolinium, adrenergic neurons against DSP-4, serotonergic neurons against 5.6-dihyroxyserotonin, and cholinergic neurons against AF64-A (for review see, for example, Ebadi *et al.*, 2002).

Regarding the neuroprotective effects of (-)-deprenyl, the key role of its enhancer effect has to be seriously considered in the future for the following reason:

The essence of the enhancer effect is that the enhancer-sensitive cell starts working on a higher activity level in the presence of an optimal concentration of a natural or a synthetic enhancer substance. Thus, whatever function of this cell is measured, the observer finds an increased activity level. It is self explanatory that if we poison the enhancer-sensitive cell, the enhancer substance will act as a protective agent. If we impair, for example, the physiological activity of an enhancer sensitive neuron in culture *via* a specific neurotoxin, the administration of a proper concentration of (-)-deprenyl or (-)-BPAP will of course protect the neuron from the deleterious effect of the neurotoxin. This protection occurs because the cell, due to the addition of the enhancer substance, works on a higher activity level. There are hundreds of papers that describe the anti-apoptotic, neuroprotective effect of (-)-deprenyl.

(-)-BPAP, at present the most potent and selective synthetic enhancer substance, is the best experimental tool to study the enhancer-sensitivity of a cell in culture to demonstrate, the dose-effect-relation characteristic to the enhancer effect. In a study performed on primary rat embryonic hippocampal cultures, we measured the protective effect of BPAP against the specific neurotoxic effect of β-amyloid$_{(25-35)}$ fraction (in this early study we worked with racemic BPAP). In this test too, BPAP exerted its effect with the same bi-modal, bell-shaped concentration effect curve as on isolated locus coerulei of rats as shown in Fig. **10**. In the presence of β-amyloid$_{(25-35)}$ fraction, the survival of the neurons decreased to 22.4±7.20% of the controls (100%), and BPAP in a concentration of 10^{-13}M (the peak of the concentration exerting the specific enhancer effect) increased the survival of the cultured neurons treated with β-amyloid$_{(25-35)}$ to 70%. BPAP also exerted a protective effect at 10^{-8}M concentration (non-specific enhancer effect) (Knoll *et al.*, 1999).

The reasonable interpretation of this finding is as follows: Whatever performance we measure in a random population, we always find a huge variation in efficiency, ranging from very low to very high performing individuals. This is also true regarding the performance of cells in a population of cultured neurons. We may look at the 20% of the cultured hippocampal neurons which survived in the presence of β-amyloid, as "high performing" cells, those possessing the most efficient BPAP-sensitive activation mechanism. Added to the cultured neurons, BPAP in the optimum concentration (10^{-13}M) is a highly potent and selective enhancer of this regulation – it made each neuron higher performing, and the survival rate increased from 20% to 70%. BPAP has obviously the same effect on the noradrenergic, dopaminergic, serotoninergic and hippocampal neurons as well. It may stimulate endogenous substances which enhance the activity of the neurons according to their physiological need. The high potency of BPAP in stimulating this regulation reasonably allows for much more potent endogenous enhancer substances than PEA and tryptamine.

As a matter of fact, up to the present, hundreds of papers confirm that enhancer-sensitive cells work on a higher activity level in presence of (-)-deprenyl, and this effect is unrelated to the MAO-B inhibitory effect of the drug. However, they ignore the fact that (-)-deprenyl acts in all these experiments as a PEA-derived synthetic enhancer substance. For example, in 1994 Tatton's group published the first study demonstrating that (-)-deprenyl reduces PC12 cell apoptosis and found that the drug induces "trophic like" rescue of dying neurons without MAO-inhibition, *since (-)-deprenyl reduced neuronal apoptosis and facilitated neuronal outgrowth in $10^{-13}M$ concentration* (Tatton *et al.*, 1994, 1995). *This is the peak in which (-)-deprenyl exerts its specific enhancer effect. Up to the present, authors mention that the observed neuroprotective effect of (-)-deprenyl is unrelated to the MAO-B inhibitory effect of the drug but neglect the fact that the mechanism through which (-)-deprenyl exerts its protective effect is already clarified.*

It is common knowledge that the activity of many important enzymes in the brain are with the passing of time on a decline and an increase in the amount of lipid peroxidation products and accumulation of lipofuscin are characteristic markers of brain aging. Kaur *et al.* measured in four brain regions (cerebral cortex, hippocampus, striatum and thalamus) the activity of sodium potassium adenosine triphosphatase (Na^+K^+-ATP-ase), glutathionperoxidase and glutathione-s-transferase, and also the levels of lipid peroxidation products and lipofuscin content in 6- and 24-month-old rats. They found an aging-related significant decline in the activities of the enzymes and a significant increase in the lipid peroxidation product and lipofuscin contents (Kaur *et al.*, 2001).

In a following study they measured the same parameters in two groups of 24-month-old rats. Prior to measurement, one group of rats was treated, intraperitoneally, for three months, with 1 mg (-)-deprenyl daily. The other group was treated with a vehicle only (control). They found that the (-)-deprenyl-treatment of aged rats significantly attenuated the aging-related-enhancement in lipid-peroxidation products and lipofuscin accumulation. The authors summarized these results as "… new additional evidence concerning the anti-aging therapeutic potential of L-deprenyl" (Kaur *et al.*, 2003). Considering the pharmacological profile of (-)-deprenyl, it is highly probable that the anti-aging effect of drug is due to its enhancer effect and is unrelated to the inhibition of B-type and/or A-type MAO. It is unfortunate that the authors used a superfluously high, 1 mg/kg dose of (-)-deprenyl, which blocks both A- and B-type MAO, instead of checking

0.001 or 0.1 mg/kg (-)-deprenyl (CAE effect) and the 0.25 mg/kg dose (selective inhibition of MAO-B).

Due to the CAE effect of (-)-deprenyl, the low dose, the chronic administration of the drug keeping the dopaminergic neurons working on a higher activity level, we expected that preventive (-)-deprenyl-treatment may protect the dopaminergic neurons from their known aging-related morphological changes. We developed a method, using a TV-image analyzer, to compare different morphological parameters in the substantia nigra of young and old male rats (Tóth *et al.*, 1992). With the aid of this method, we determined the number, total area, area of one granule, and density features (sum and average of gray values and average gray value of one pigment granule) of melanin granules in neurocytes of the substantia nigra in 3-month-old and 21-month-old male rats (Knoll *et al.*, 1992b).

Within the melanin-containing neurocytes, we discovered statistically significant aging-related differences in the number, area, and density features of melanin granules. Whereas in the young rats the majority of the neurocytes contained numerous, small-sized neuromelanin granules, the majority of the neurocytes of old rats, smaller numbers of large-sized neuromelanin granules were detected. We treated rats subcutaneously, three times a week with 0.25 mg/kg (-)-deprenyl for 18 months and found that this treatment prevented the aging-related morphological changes in the neurocytes of the substantia nigra. This was *prima facie* morphological evidence for the anti-aging effect of prophylactic treatment with a synthetic enhancer substance (Knoll *et al.*, 1992b).

Rinne *et al.* (1991) found that the number of medial nigral neurons was greater and the number of Lewy bodies fewer in patients with PD who had been treated with (-)-deprenyl in combination with levodopa when compared with patients who had received levodopa alone. Lewy bodies are composed mainly of α-synuclein. In a recent study, Braga *et al.* evaluated the effects of (-)-deprenyl on the *in vitro* aggregation of a type of α-synuclein and found that (-)-deprenyl delays fibril formation by extending the lag phase of aggregation. They showed that in the presence of (-)-deprenyl, electron microscopy reveals amorphous heterogeneous aggregates, including large annular species, which are innocuous to a primary culture enriched in dopaminergic neurons while their age-matched counterparts are toxic. They also found that (-)-deprenyl blocks the formation of smaller toxic aggregates by perturbing dopamine-dependent fibril disaggregation. Thus, (-)-deprenyl slows the fibrillation, giving rise to the formation of large nontoxic aggregates. They concluded that "These effects might be beneficial for PD patients, since the sequestration of protofibrils into fibrils or the inhibition of fibril dissociation could alleviate the toxic effect of protofibrils on dopaminergic neurons. Selegiline might slow the fibrillation, giving rise to the formation of large nontoxic aggregates" (Braga *et al.*, 2011).

By now dozens of papers are published in literature demonstrating that low concentrations (10^{-8} - 10^{-15}M) changed significantly the activity of isolated cells in culture, clearly demonstrating that the authors detected the enhancer-effect of the drug, thus proved that they worked on an enhancer sensitive cell. For example, Esmaeili *et al.* published in 2006 that they worked with the mouse embryonic stem cell line CCE, and found that selegiline induced, with a peak at 10^{-8}M, neuronal differentiation in the undifferentiated pluripotent embryonic stem cells and the authors suggested to use combined selegiline and stem cell therapy to improve deficits in neurodegenerative diseases in aging (Esmaeili *et al.*, 2006).

In a similar publication in 2011 a work was carried out with the P19 line of murine embryonal carcinoma (EC) stem cells. Embryonal carcinoma cells, like embryonic stem cells, on which the formal study was done, are developmentally pluripotent cells which can differentiate into all cell types under appropriate conditions. They investigated the effect of selegiline on undifferentiated P19 line of murine EC stem cells and found that selegiline had a dramatic effect on neuronal morphology. Selegiline induced in low concentrations (10^{-8} - 10^{-10}M) the differentiation of EC cells into neuron-like cells (Bakshalizadeh *et al.*, 2011).

Despite the convincing experimental evidence that selegiline in low concentrations acts as a PEA-derived synthetic CAE substance, and the results published in both papers furnish unequivocal evidence that both the mouse embryonic stem cells and the embryonic carcinoma cells are enhancer-sensitive cells, the authors of the two papers cited altogether three of my papers written in 1983, 1985 and 1988, thus prior to the discovery of the enhancer-regulation in the brain.

CHAPTER 5

The Age-Related Decline of Dopaminergic Activity and the Reason Why Low Dose of (-)-Deprenyl Slows Brain Aging and Prolongs Life

Aging, the unfortunate common fate of all mature adults, is a physiological phenomenon. It essentially means the decadence of the quality of life with the passage of time. The easily recognizable, external appearance of aging (graying hair, wrinkling skin, use of reading glasses, *etc.*) gives some information about the chronological age of the person, but these signs are not necessarily in complete harmony with the physiological age of the organ systems, with the measurable decrements of integrated functions (maximum O_2 capacity, maximum breathing capacity, maximum work rate, *etc.*) or with the almost immeasurable mental deterioration.

The exact measurement of the aging-related changes in man remains difficult because the most reliable technique for following the changes in a given individual over his or her entire lifespan is practically unfeasible. The available information about the aging-related changes in human population stems from cross-sectional studies, from the comparison of differences in performances between different age-groups.

The main problem is, however, that the scatter within a particular age-group for any measurable parameter is extreme. The reason for this extreme variation is the lack of a general factor of physiological age. In cross-sectional studies no single age emerges as the point of sharp decline in function. Any individual may show different levels of performance and the careful observer finds much dissociation between "chronological" and "physiological" age. Despite of all these weaknesses, the average lifespan in most developed countries has already exceeded the 80-year average. This change has come about due to the prevention of premature deaths through the development of hygiene, immunology and chemotherapy. The technical lifespan of the human race (TLS$_h$), close to 120 years, has remained, however, unchanged.

Since the catecholaminergic and serotonergic neurons in the brain stem are of key importance in ensuring that the mammalian organism works as a purposeful, motivated, goal-directed entity, it is hard to overestimate the significance of finding safe and efficient means to slow the decay of these systems with passing time. The conclusion that the maintenance on (-)-deprenyl that keeps the catecholaminergic neurons on a higher activity level is a safe and efficient anti-aging therapy follows from the discovery of the enhancer regulation in the catecholaminergic neurons of the brain stem. From the finding that this regulation starts working on a high activity level after weaning and the enhanced activity subsists during the uphill period of life, until sexual hormones dampen the enhancer regulation in the catecholaminergic and serotonergic neurons in the brain stem, and this event signifies the transition from developmental longevity into postdevelopmental longevity, the downhill period of life.

Since the dopaminergic system is the most rapidly aging, life's important machinery in the human brain, the possibility to slow the aging of these group of neurons by the continuous daily administration of a small amount of (-)-deprenyl during the postdevelopmental phase of life, from sexual maturity until death, is by now the best example of a firmly based physiologically and pharmacologically safe anti-aging therapy with a significant promise of efficiency. The aging of the dopaminergic system means that with the passing of time the amount of dopamine, the transmitter of the system, and PEA, the modulator of the system, an important natural enhancer substance, is on a continuous decline.

PEA, like tryptamine, p-tyramine, m-tyramine, and octopamine, belongs to the trace amines, the family of endogenous amines present in the mammalian CNS in trace amounts (Usdin & Sandler, 1976). PEA, to date probably the most carefully investigated trace amine is, like tryptamine, a natural enhancer substance (see Knoll, 2005, Sect.3.1.2.). The first note in literature furnishing indirect evidence that PEA may be an endogenous CNS stimulant in humans was the finding of Fischer *et al.,* (1968). They found that the urinary excretion of free PEA was reduced in depressed patients and suggested that a PEA deficit may be one of the biochemical lesions leading to depression. Experimental evidence, soon presented that PEA is an endogenous constituent of the mammalian brain (Fischer *et al.,* 1972; Saavedra, 1974; Wilner *et al.,* 1974).

Sabelli & Mosnaim (1974) expounded the hypothesis that PEA might play a physiological role in effective behavior. Thereafter, papers discussing the possible role of PEA as a physiological mood elevator (Greenshow, 1989; Davis & Boulton, 1994; Sabelli & Javaid, 1995; Sabelli *et al.*, 1986; Premont *et al.*, 2001), as well as, papers proposing a role of trace-amines in a series of illnesses, such as schizophrenia, depression, attention deficit/hyperactive disorder, PD, Rett's syndrome, migraine, phenylketonuria, hepatic encephalopathy, and hypertension (Usdin & Sandler, 1976; Boulton *et al.*, 1988; Saavedra, 1989; Walker *et al.*, 1996; Janssen *et al.*, 1999; Satoi *et al.*, 2000; Premont *et al.*, 2001) were continually published.

An important step forward in the history of trace-amines was the discovery of the presence of high-affinity binding sites for tyramine, tryptamine, and PEA (Hauger *et al.*, 1982; Nguyen & Juorio, 1989; Nguyen *et al.*, 1989). The trace-amine binding sites have been identified as G-protein-coupled receptors (GPCRs) (see Knoll, 2005, Sect. 3.3.). The expression of trace-amine receptor mRNA in the human amygdala further suggests a role of trace-amines in depression and anxiety disorders (Borowsky *et al.*, 2001); and methamphetamine, the PEA-derivative with a long-lasting effect, is also a trace-amine receptor agonist (Bunzow *et al.*, 2001). The identification of members of the GPCR family in human, chimpanzee, rat and mouse showed remarkable interspecies differences, even between human and chimpanzee. Most of the receptors do not respond to trace amines. So far a clear functional relationship between some trace amines and trace amine receptors has been established only for two members (TA receptors 1 and 2) (Lindemann *et al.*, 2005). It remains for future research to find the relationship between our synthetic enhancer substances and TA receptors.

The discovery that PEA is a natural enhancer substance clarified the mechanism of the stimulatory effect of PEA and finally assigned the physiological role of this trace-amine in the regulation of behavioral performances (see Shimazu & Miklya, 2004, for review). Long before the discovery of the enhancer effect of PEA (Knoll *et al.*, 1996c), we had already established that during postdevelopmental longevity there is a continuously increasing PEA deficit in the mammalian brain (Knoll, 1982). The thesis of this paper put forth that the progressive decrease in brain catecholamines and trace-amines is an unavoidable biochemical lesion of aging.

This concept was based, on the one hand, on the enhanced MAO-B activity in the aging brain, and on the other hand, on the anti-aging effect of (-)-deprenyl, the first described highly potent and selective inhibitor of MAO-B.

As a rule, enzyme functions decrease in the brain with the passing of time. B-type of MAO is an exception. Robinson *et al.,* (1971, 1972) published the first papers demonstrating that MAO activity progressively increases in the aging brain. This finding was corroborated within a couple of years by different groups (Nies *et al.,* 1973; Mantle *et al.,* 1976; Shih, 1979; Carlsson, 1979; Eckert *et al.,* 1980; Fowler *et al.,* 1980a,b; Strolin Benedetti & Keane, 1980). It soon became clear, however, that in both the human (Fowler *et al.,* 1980b) and rat (Mantle *et al.,* 1976; Strolin Benedetti & Keane, 1980) brains only the activity of MAO-B is increased in the aged. It was also shown that the selective age-dependent decrease in MAO-B activity was due entirely to an increased enzyme concentration in brain tissue (Fowler *et al.,* 1980b). Student & Edwards (1977) demonstrated that MAO-B is predominantly localized in the neuroglia, a finding soon corroborated (Strolin Benedetti & Keane, 1980) and now firmly established as fact.

In my hypothesis put forth in 1981-1982, I suggested that a progressively developing catecholaminergic and trace-aminergic deficiency is the biochemical lesion in the aging brain which leads to the age-related decline in sexual and learning performances and ultimately leads to natural death (Knoll, 1981a,b,c, 1982).

Let us quote here the original description of the hypothesis (Knoll, 1982, pp.109-110):

Well established old experiences offer a good explanation for the increase of brain MAO-B activity in the latter decades of life. Cell loss is a general feature of the aging brain.As the loss of neurons is always compensated by glial cells, the progressive and cumulative loss of neurons in the aging brain gives a satisfactory explanation to the selective increase of extrasynaptosomal MAO-B activity with increasing age. This seems to be an unavoidable biochemical lesion of aging. Collating the facts that there is an unavoidable loss of neurons, inescapably leading to increased MAO-B activity with increasing age, makes it understandable that dopaminergic and trace-aminergic modulation in the brain is progressively decreasing in the aging brain. It is in agreement with this trend of changes that an age-dependent decrease in the dopamine control of the basal ganglia in man was described, first by Bertler (1961), and corroborated by many others. Riederer and Wuketich (1976) found that the dopamine content of the human caudate nucleus decreased in an age-related manner.

If, in addition, we also consider that the activity of tyrosine hydroxylase, the enzyme catalysing the rate-limiting step in catecholamine biosynthesis, was also found to decrease in human brain tissue with increasing age (McGeer *et al.*, 1971), weighty arguments seem to support the view that catecholaminergic tone is progressively decreasing in the aging brain.

As the described age-dependent chain of events can be deduced to well defined biochemical lesions, the chances to develop a new drug strategy for counteracting or possibly even preventing, the adverse consequences of the age-related decrease of the catecholaminergic tone in the brain, are fair.

Dozens of studies published since the proposal of this hypothesis strengthened this approach step-by-step. The evolution of the project can be followed *via* the reviews published after 1982, when the original hypothesis was presented, until the discovery of the enhancer regulation in the brain stem neurons (Knoll, 1983, 1985, 1986a,b,c, 1989, 1992a,b, 1993a,b,c, 1995, 1998, 2001, 2003).

In the light of our present knowledge there can be little doubt that because of the continuously increasing MAO-B activity in the aging brain, the more and more efficient metabolism of PEA, necessarily works against the chances of a freshly synthesized PEA molecule reaching its target. This is obviously a significant factor which contributes to the aging-related decline of the enhancer regulation in the catecholaminergic brain engine with the passing of time.

The same decline applies to dopamine. Fig. **17** shows the decay in the dopamine content of the caudate nucleus in the aging human brain. We lose 13% of our brain dopamine in the decade after age 45. At this normal rate, nobody will exceed, within the obtainable human lifespan the critical threshold of the dopamine content (30%) that accompanies the precipitation of the symptoms of PD. Thus, as illustrated in Fig. **17**, PD is obviously the consequence of a premature aging of the dopaminergic machinery in the human brain.

THE AGE-RELATED DECLINE OF STRIATAL DOPAMINE IN HUMANS

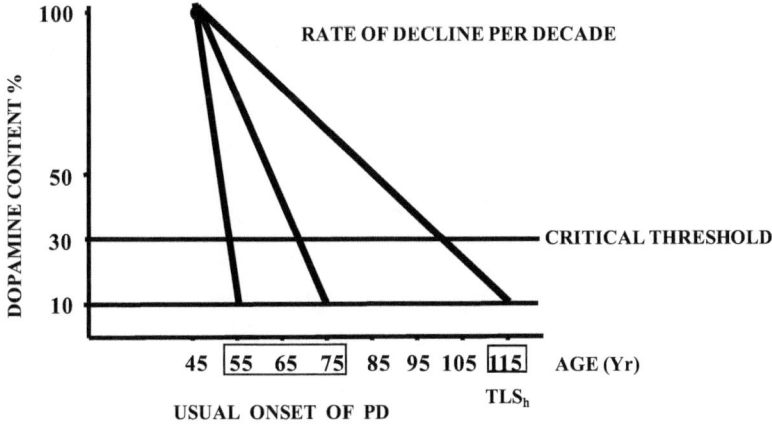

Figure 17: Visualization of the concept that PD is the premature rapid aging of the striatal dopaminergic machinery. TLS_h: technical lifespan in humans.

To realize the functional consequences of the aging-related decline of the dopaminergic system in the mesencephalon, let us follow, as an example, the decline of the ejaculatory activity in human and rat males during their postdevelopmental phase of life.

Sexual activity in the human male is known to be influenced by a number of factors, such as good health, stable marriage, satisfactory sexual partner(s), and adequate financial and social status. But even in the males who meet all the requirements for retention and maintenance of sexual functioning, there is an age-related decrease in sexual vigor.

In the Baltimore Longitudinal Study of Aging, coital activity was studied as function of age. They interviewed 628 members of the Washington-Baltimore area, varying from 20-95 years of age, white, married, urban residents in good health. According to this study the median coital activity was highest, 2.1 events/week, between ages of 30-34, and decreased progressively with increasing age, sinking to 0.2/week in the age-group 65-69.

It is common knowledge that individual variation in sexual vigor is enormous. In this study the mean frequency of total sexual activity in 159 males was found to be 520 sexual events/5 years in the age-group 20-39, including young males performing below 100 sexual events/5 years and those with frequencies of total sexual activity over 1000 sexual events/5 years. In the age-group 65-79, the mean frequency of total sexual activity decreased to 75 sexual events/5 years, but even in this group subjects producing 400-700 sexual events/5 years were registered (Martin, 1977).

In a number of longitudinal studies performed on male rats we observed that the age-related decline of coital activity in male rats and the striking individual differences in sexual performance in different age cohorts are essentially the same as in human males (Knoll, 1988, 1989; Knoll *et al.*, 1983, 1994).

Because of brain aging, even the most sexually high performing males may lose their potency to ejaculate if they live long enough. In our studies on male CFY rats, we followed the sexual performance of the animals once a week from sexual maturity until death. We measured three patterns: mounting, intromission, and ejaculation. We found that in response to brain aging even the best performing individuals lost their potency to ejaculate not later than at the completion of their second year of age (Knoll *et al.*, 1983).

The results of our first longevity study (Knoll, 1988, Knoll *et al.*, 1989) clearly proved in retrospect that the age-related decline of the sexual performance of male rats signals the decay of the enhancer regulation in the dopaminergic neurons with the passing of time.

As already discussed in Chapter 2, in this series of experiments, we selected 132 aged, *2-year-old* male rats and measured in four consecutive, weekly mating tests their sexual performance: mounting, intromission and ejaculation. Due to aging, the ability to ejaculate was not longer detectable in 2-year-old CFY rats. We classified the rats according to their sexual performance in the testing period as noncopulators (no sign of sexual activity), mounting rats (displayed mounting only), and sluggish rats (displayed mounting and intromission). Of the 132 rats 46 were found to be noncopulators (Group 1), 42 displayed mounting only (Group 2), and 44 rats proved to be sluggish (Group 3). After the selection period, we started to treat half of the rats with saline (1 ml/kg) and half with (-)-deprenyl (0.25

mg/kg) three times a week, until they died. We tested their sexual performance once a week. The dying out of the 66 saline-treated rats showed that lifespan was inversely proportional to their sexual performance (see Table VI in Knoll, 1988).

As sexual performance is directly proportional to the functional state of the enhancer regulation in the dopaminergic neurons, we assume that rats die when the age-related decline in mesencephalic enhancer regulation arrives to a critical threshold. With regard to sexual performance: Group 1 < Group 2 < Group 3, thus, rats belonging to Group 1 are the closest to exceeding the critical threshold resulting in natural death and die out first, rats in Group 2 live longer, and rats in Group 3 live the longest.

The age-related decline in mesencephalic enhancer regulation during the postdevelopmental phase of life in male rats can be further recognized by comparing the individual variation in sexual performance of 3-6-month-old male rats with the performance of their 2-year-old peers. Whereas 52.49% of 3-6-month-old male rats displayed ejaculations during the four consecutive mating tests, only 5.80% of 12-18-month-old males ejaculated, and none of the 24-month-old males were in possession of this faculty any longer (see Table 3.5. in Knoll, 2005).

Moreover, the age-related change in the percentage of animals belonging to the "non-copulator" group clearly proved that enhancer regulation in the dopaminergic neurons is in continuous decline during the postdevelopmental phase of life. Only 5.51% of the 3-6-month-old males were sexually inactive, but 19.56% of the 12-18-month-old rats and 34.84% of the 24-month-old rats belonged to this group.

Due to the striking similarities between human and rat males in the age-related decline of their sexual activity it is hard to deny that the decay of the dopaminergic machinery with the passing of time plays the key role on the final loss of the ability to ejaculate, from which there is no escape. We demonstrated with a series of experiments that the treatment of male rats with (-)-deprenyl significantly enhanced their sexual activity and with the preventive administration of a small dose of (-)-deprenyl the loss of the ability to ejaculate was substantially shifted in time (Knoll, 1988, 1989, 1990, 1993a; Knoll *et al.*, 1983, 1989, 1994; Yen *et al.*, 1982).

Table **8**, a brief summary of the results of our first longevity study, shows that the anti-aging effect of (-)-deprenyl was decisive even in a series of experiments performed on two-year-old rats which had already lost their ability to ejaculate.

Table 8: Illustration of the antiaging effect of (-)-deprenyl treatment. Data taken from Knoll, 1989, Table IV. Details explained in text

Classification of the Groups According to Sexual Performance Before Treatment	Number of Animals	Total Number of Mountings (M), Intromissions (I) and Ejaculations (E) of the Groups During Treatment		
		M	I	E
		Saline-Treated Rats		
Non-copulators	23	37	0	0
Mounting rats	21	425	54	0
Sluggish rats	22	477	231	0
		(-)-Deprenyl-Treated Rats		
Non-copulators	23	997	544	190
Mounting rats	21	1129	662	172
Sluggish rats	22	1696	1257	481

A second example is an experiment performed on young male CFY rats. We selected 90 males possessing full-scale sexual activity. Half of the population was treated with saline (1 ml/kg), the other half with (-)-deprenyl (0.25 mg/kg), three times a week, from the 25th week of age. The rats' sexual performance was tested once a week. In this study, the loss in the ability to ejaculate was selected as the age-related end stage. Saline-treated rats reached this stage at an average of 112±9 weeks. In contrast, (-)-deprenyl-treated rats reached it at an average of 150±12 weeks ($P<0.001$) (Fig. **2** in Knoll, 1993a). As sexual performance is a dopaminergic function, it became obvious that the enhanced activity of the mesencephalic dopaminergic neurons was responsible for the significantly retarded loss of the ability to ejaculate in the (-)-deprenyl-treated group.

Our finding that (-)-deprenyl prolongs life was confirmed in rats, mice, hamsters, and dogs, even on a fly (*Drosophila melanogaster*), widely used as an experimental model of aging (Table **9**).

Table 9: Our longevity studies and the confirmation of the finding (m - male; f –female).

YEAR		SPECIES	CONFIRMATION	SPECIES
1988	Knoll J	Wistar Logan Rats (m)		
1989	Knoll, Dalló, Yen;	Wistar Logan Rats (m)		
1990			Milgram *et al.*	Fischer 344 Rats (m)
1993			Kitani *et al.*	F 344 Rats (m)
1994	Knoll, Yen, Miklya	Wistar Logan Rats (m)	Freisleben *et al.*	Mice (m)
1996	Dalló, Köles	Wistar Logan Rats (f)	Archer & Harrison	Mice (m, f)
1997			Stoll *et al.* Ruehl et al Bickford *et al.*	Syrian hamster (f) Beagle dogs F344 rats (m)
1999			Jordens *et al.*	*Drosophila melanogaster*

In one strain of mice (-)-deprenyl-treatment had no beneficial effect on survival (Ingram *et al.*, 1993); and Stoll *et al.,* (1997) found increased lifespan in (-)-deprenyl-treated female hamsters only. Moreover, in the longevity studies substantial strain differences were found in the efficiency of (-)-deprenyl. It has to be considered, however, that enhancer substances stimulate the enhancer-sensitive neurons in the brain stem in a peculiar manner (see Fig. **10**). Thus, the same dose of an enhancer drug may exert a peak effect on one strain, a much lower effect on an other strain, and be ineffective on a third strain.

This problem was analyzed in a whole series of papers (for review see Miklya, 2011). Kitani *et al.*, working with F344 rats, found for example that 0.25 mg/kg (-)-deprenyl significantly prolonged in this strain the lifespan of both male and female rats whereas a greater dose became less effective and may actually adversely effect the lifespan of rats (Kitani *et al.*, 2005). Leaving aside these pecualiarities, authors may easily fail to observe the beneficial effect of (-)-deprenyl treatment upon longevity.

Nevertheless, even from a study with the conclusion that a clear effect of chronic (-)-deprenyl treatment upon longevity was not observed, a closer examination of the published data shows the beneficial effect of (-)-deprenyl on the survival of rats. For example, Bickford *et al.,* (1997) treated the short living male F344 rats with (-)-deprenyl. Beginning at 54 weeks of age, the drug was administered *via* drinking water containing 8 µg (-)-deprenyl/ml. The estimated daily dose of (-)-deprenyl was 0.5 mg/kg. After 64 weeks of (-)-deprenyl treatment, MAO-B activity in the striatum, hippocampus and cerebellum were reduced by 85 to 88 % and MAO-A activity remained unchanged. This study proved that drinking water was an effective method for the delivery of (-)-deprenyl. The authors measured at 84 weeks of age sensorimotor skills, at 86 weeks motor learning, at 104 weeks spatial learning and at 118 weeks they performed quantitative receptor autoradiography. According to their final conclusion "… long term oral administration of (-)-deprenyl extended the functional lifespan of rats with respect to cognitive, but not motor performance". The survival curves in their study (Fig. **1**) reveal that in comparison to the controls, the (-)-deprenyl-treated rats exhibited higher survival rates at all points after 63 weeks of age. The maximum difference in survival rates, about 20%, between the population of (-)-deprenyl-treated and control rats, was reached between approximately 100-108 weeks of age.

As shown in Chapter 2, (-)-deprenyl is a potent enhancer of the catecholaminergic neurons in brain stem. In AD and PD, neuronal loss in the locus coeruleus was found to be even greater than in the substantia nigra (Zarow *et al.*, 2003). More recent data supports that aging of the noradrenergic system in the brain plays an important role in the manifestation of neurodegenerative diseases, such as PD and AD, and enhanced noradrenergic activity might substantially contribute to (-)-deprenyl-treatment-induced slowing of the age-related decline of brain functions (for review see Miklya, 2011).

Send Orders of Reprints at reprints@benthamscience.org

CHAPTER 6

Benefits of Selegiline in the Treatment of Parkinson's Disease (PD)

As discussed in Chapter 1, in order to lessen the serious side effects of levodopa-treatment in PD, Birkmayer and Hornykiewicz tried to achieve a levodopa-sparing effect by the concurrent administration of levodopa with an MAO-inhibitor. They were compelled to terminate this trial because the combination elicited hypertensive attacks. Since selegiline was the unique MAO inhibitor free of the cheese effect, Birkmayer dared to combine selegiline with levodopa, and a levodopa-sparing effect was achieved in patients without side effects (Birkmayer *et al.*, 1977). The levodopa-sparing effect of selegiline is fully related to the selective inhibition of B-type MAO.

The safety profile of daily 10 mg dose of selegiline, given regularly in the treatment of PD, is favorable (Heinonen, 1998). The usually mild side effects (dry mouth, anxiety, sleep disturbances, confusion, nausea, dizziness, orthostatic hypotension, and hallucination) are rare (for review see Robottom, 2011). Patients taking nonselective MAO inhibitors in combination with selective serotonin reuptake inhibitors (SSRIs) may develop quite dangerous serotonin syndrome, but there is no significant interaction between fluoxetin and selegiline (Waters, 1994).

As a matter of fact, it was the DATATOP study's results that selegiline has a beneficial influence on the natural history of PD, which clearly proved that the CAE effect of selegiline is fully responsible for this unique benefit. Although the Parkinson Study Group organized the DATATOP study with the belief that selegiline will act beneficially in this multicenter clinical trial because it inhibits selectively MAO-B, the outcome presented clear-cut evidence that the CAE effect of selegiline was fully responsible in changing the course of the disease in *de novo* parkinsonians in a unique beneficial manner.

It is remarkable that despite the unequivocal experimental evidence, the fact that selegiline is primarily a PEA-derived CAE substance is ignored. Today, clinicians still classify selegiline, at present the only synthetic CAE substance in clinical use, as merely a selective inhibitor of B-type MAO. Lazabemide, after selegiline the second selective inhibitor of MAO-B in clinical use, is devoid of the enhancer effect (Miklya & Knoll, 2003, see also Chapter 9). The same fits for rasagiline, the recently introduced third selective inhibitor of MAO-B in clinical use (Miklya, 2011). It is reasonable to draw a parallel in this respect from the DATATOP study.

As was discussed in detail earlier, convincing animal experiments speak in favor for the conclusion that selegiline slows the rate of the functional deterioration of the nigrostriatal dopaminergic neurones, and the experimental findings are in harmony with clinical evidence that selegiline slows the progress of PD. The indication for using selegiline in patients with early, untreated PD was established in the DATATOP study in the USA (Tetrud & Langston, 1989; Parkinson Study Group, 1989, 1993). Important multicenter studies such as, the French Selegiline Multicenter Trial (FSMT) (Allain *et al.*, 1991), the Finnish Study (Myttyla *et al.*, 1992), the Swedish Parkinson Study Group (Palhagen *et al.,* 1998), and the Norwegian-Danish Study Group (Larsen *et al.*, 1999) confirmed the usefulness of the drug in *de novo* PD.

Age-related deterioration of the striatal machinery is a continuum and any precisely determined short segment of it is sufficient to measure the rate of decline in the presence or absence of selegiline. As a matter of fact, in the DATATOP multicenter study by the Parkinson Study Group, a segment of this continuum, the time elapsing from diagnosis of PD until levodopa was needed, was properly measured in untreated patients with PD and the effect of selegiline *versus* placebo was compared (Parkinson Study Group, 1989). It is common experience that it belongs to the natural history of PD that due to the continuous further deterioration of the nigrostriatal dopaminergic neurons usually within one year after the diagnosis of the disease the patients need dopamine-substitution (levodopa therapy). Among the participants of the DATATOP multicenter study Tetrud and Langston were the first who realized that selegiline-treatment affects beneficially the natural history of PD. In 1989 they published that selegiline delays the need for levodopa therapy. In their study, the average time that elapsed before levodopa was needed was 312.1 days for patients in the placebo group and 548.9 days for patients in the selegiline group (Tetrud & Langston, 1989). This was clear proof that selegiline, which enhances the activity of the surviving dopaminergic neurons, kept these neurons on a higher activity level for a longer duration of time.

The design of the DATATOP study was unintentionally similar that we had used in our rat experiments with (-)-deprenyl since 1980. We tested the sexual activity of male rats as a quantitatively measurable, rapidly aging dopaminergic function, and compared the effect of (-)-deprenyl *versus* saline treatment on the age-related decline of copulatory activity in rats. We demonstrated that (-)-deprenyl treatment significantly slowed the age-related decay of sexual performance (Knoll, 1982) and later went on to show that this effect of (-)-deprenyl was unrelated to the inhibition of MAO-B. We performed a structure-activity-relationship study which aimed to select a derivative of (-)-deprenyl that was free of any MAO inhibitory property (Knoll *et al.*, 1992a). In (-)-deprenyl, the propargyl group covalently bonded to the flavin of MAO-B, and this led to the irreversible inhibition of the enzyme activity. (-)-1-Phenyl-2-propylaminopentane [(-)-PPAP], the new (-)-deprenyl analogue selected, differed from its mother compound by containing a propyl group instead of a propargyl group. As expected, this compound enhanced dopaminergic activity in the brain like (-)-deprenyl, but did not change the activity of MAO-B. One can follow the progress in clarifying the mechanism in (-)-deprenyl responsible for enhanced dopaminergic activity by referring to a series of reviews (Knoll, 1978, 1983, 1987, 1992 a, b, 1995, 1998, 2001, 2003).

By now, it is clear that if we select a quantitatively measurable dopaminergic function and determine its age-related decline by fixing an exact end, there is a shift of this end stage in time in (-)-deprenyl-treated rats which shows the dopaminergic activity enhancer effect of the drug. For example, due primarily to the physiological aging of the striatal dopaminergic system, male rats ultimately lose their ability to ejaculate. As already reviewed in Chapter 5, we found that saline-treated Charles River rats reached this stage at the age of 112 ± 9 weeks, whereas their (-)-deprenyl-treated peers lost the ability to ejaculate only at the age of 150 ± 12 weeks ($P < 0.001$) (Knoll, 1993a).

The design of the DATATOP study was essentially the same. The authors knew that after having diagnosed PD the next step would be the need for levodopa, and they measured the selegiline-induced delay in reaching this stage.

The authors of the DATATOP study expected selegiline to be efficient in their trial because of its MAO-B inhibitory effect. Their hypothesis was that the activity of MAO and the formation of free radicals predispose patients to nigral degeneration and contribute to the emergence and progression of PD. In accord with their working hypothesis they expected that selegiline, the MAO inhibitor, α-tocopherol, the antioxidant, and the combination of the two compounds will slow the clinical progression of the disease because MAO activity and the formation of oxygen radicals contribute to the pathogenesis of nigral degeneration. They selected patients with early, untreated PD and measured the delay in the onset of disability necessitating levodopa therapy.

In the first phase of the trial, 401 subjects were assigned to α-tocopherol or placebo and 399 subjects were assigned to selegiline, alone or with α-tocopherol. Only 97 subjects who received selegiline reached the 'end' of the trial (*i.e.,* the onset of disability necessitating levodopa therapy) during an average 12 months of follow-up compared with 176 subjects who did not receive selegiline. The risk of reaching the end of the trial was reduced by 57% for the subject who received selegiline, and these patients also had a significant reduction in their risk of having to give up full-time employment (Parkinson Study Group, 1989). Following the course of changes, the authors concluded in their next paper (Parkinson Study Group, 1993) that selegiline, but not α-tocopherol, delayed the onset of disability associated with early, otherwise untreated PD. But as time passed, the DATATOP study also revealed that selegiline did not reduce the occurrence of subsequent levodopa-associated adverse effects in the patients (Parkinson Study Group, 1996).

The unexpected outcome of the DATATOP study clearly indicated that selegiline possesses an unknown pharmacological effect of basic importance and α-tocopherol is devoid of this effect. We succeeded in the 1990s to explain the ineffectiveness of α-tocopherol in the DATATOP study. As shown in detail earlier, we demonstrated that PEA and tyramine are not only well-known releasers of catecholamines from their intraneuronal pools, but they are primarily CAE substances. They enhance in low doses the impulse propagation mediated release of catecholamines. Since the catecholamine-releasing property of these amines concealed the CAE effect, the physiologically important property of these amines remained undetected (Knoll *et al.*, 1996c). As expected, a comparison of the enhancer effect of α-tocopherol with that of (-)-deprenyl showed that α-tocopherol did not change the impulse-evoked release of norepinephrine, dopamine and serotonin in the brain; thus it is devoid of an enhancer effect (Miklya *et al.*, 2003). This is clear proof that the CAE effect was responsible for the effectiveness of selegiline in the DATATOP study (as a recent review see Miklya, 2011). The clinical trial with rasagiline, performed by the Parkinson Study Group, revealed that unlike the early selegiline trials, rasagiline failed to demonstrate a decreased need for levodopa (Parkinson Study Group, 2002). Even the results of a couple of recent studies (Olanow & Rascol, 2010; Ahlskog and Uitti, 2010; Mehta *et al.*, 2010) led to the conclusion that "based on current evidence, rasagiline cannot be said to definitely have a disease-modifying effect" (Robottom, 2011).

We have to consider the physiological role of the nigrostriatal dopaminergic neurons in the continuous activation of the cerebral cortex. This is realized *via* a highly complicated route of connections. The neostriatum is the main input structure of the basal ganglia. It gets glutamatergic input from many areas of the cerebral cortex. Cholinergic and peptidergic striatal interneurons are in connection with the nigrostriatal dopaminergic neurons. Dopamine released in the striatum controls the two GABAergic pathways along which the outflow of the striatum proceeds. One is a direct route to the substantia nigra pars compacta and medial globus pallidus. The other is an indirect route. A GABAergic link binds the striatum to the lateral globus pallidus; from here, another GABAergic pathway goes to the subthalamic nucleus, which provides glutamatergic excitatory innervation to the substantia nigra pars compacta and medial globus pallidus. This then continuously inhibits - *via* a GABAergic projection - the activity of the ventroanterior and ventrolateral nuclei of the thalamus, which provide feedback glutamatergic excitatory impulses to the cerebral cortex.

Thus, the stimulation of the direct pathway at the level of the striatum increases the excitatory outflow from the thalamus to the cortex, whereas stimulation of the indirect pathway has the opposite effect. The striatal GABAergic neurons of the direct pathway express primarily the excitatory D_1 dopamine receptors; the striatal neurons of the indirect pathway express primarily the inhibitory D_2 receptors. As a result, dopamine release in the striatum increases the inhibitory activity of the direct pathway and diminishes the excitatory activity of the indirect pathway. As a net effect, the inhibitory influence of the substantia nigra pars reticulata and medial globus pallidus on the ventroanterior and ventrolateral nuclei of the thalamus is reduced, thus increasing the excitatory effect of these nuclei on the cerebral cortex. All in all, *a more active nigrostriatal dopaminergic system means a more active cerebral cortex and, vice versa.* The physiological age-related decline of the nigrostriatal dopaminergic activity leads to an equivalent reduction in the activity of the cerebral cortex. It is reasonable to conclude that the age-related decline of the nigrostriatal dopaminergic brain mechanism plays a significant role in the decline of performances over time.

Aging of the dopaminergic system in the brain plays an undisputable leading role in the highly significant, substantial decline in male sexual activity and also in the more modest but still significant age-related decline in learning performance. As discussed in Chapter 5, in a human male study median coital activity was the highest, 2.1 events/week, between the ages of 30 and 34. This rate decreased progressively with increasing age, sinking to 0.2/week ($P<0.001$) in the 65- to 69-year-old age group. We found essentially the same trend of changes in male rats in a series of different experiments.

There is a quantitative difference only between the physiological age-related decline of the dopaminergic input and that observed in PD. In the healthy population, the calculated loss of striatal dopamine is about 40% at the age of 75, which is about the average lifetime. The loss of dopamine in PD is 70% or thereabout at diagnosis and over 90% at death. The drastic reduction of the dopaminergic output in PD evidently leads to an accordingly drastic reduction of cortical activity and *this makes it clear why an enhancer substance, like (-)-deprenyl, improves cognition, attention, memory and reaction times. It also brings about subjective feelings of increased vitality, euphoria and increased energy in people with PD.*

In diagnosing PD, the neurologist selects subjects with the most rapidly aging striatal dopaminergic system (about 0.1% of the population). As symptoms of PD become visible only after the unnoticed loss of a major part (about 70%) of striatal dopamine and further deterioration is irresistible, the disease is, in this sense, incurable.

It is obvious that with the progression of the disease the chances to enhance the activity of the dopaminergic neurons *via* the administration of a synthetic enhancer substance are going from bad to worse. PD is, after all, an incurable disease. In a recent study the clinical outcome of PD patients treated with selegiline plus levodopa was evaluated in the early stage of the disease in comparison with that of late-stage use of only selegiline. The clinical outcome, as evaluated by the selected Unified PD Rating Scale (UPDRS) motor scores was better for levodopa-treated patients who received selegiline within 5 years from the onset compared with those who received selegiline approximately 10 years from the onset (Mizuno *et al.*, 2010). On the other hand, a recent study confirmed even that patients who were treated with selegiline for 3 or more years in early PD showed a slower progression of the disease, as evaluated by the Hoen and Yahr Stage transition times (Zhao *et al.*, 2011).

Prevention is the only chance to fight off PD. We need to start slowing the age-related functional decline of the mesencephalic enhancer regulation in due time. For this reason it is advisable to begin the preventive administration of a synthetic enhancer substance, for example 1 mg selegiline/day, as soon as sexual maturity has been reached and the postdevelopmental period of life has just started. It is therefore of particular importance that selegiline, to date the only synthetic enhancer substance in clinical use, has proven to be an unusually safe drug (see further analysis in Chapter 9).

Due to the inhibition of MAO-B, selegiline treatment allows for a 20-50% decrease in levodopa dose needed in PD. In patients who need levodopa, however, there is always a risk that the administration of selegiline will enhance the side effects of levodopa which can only be avoided by properly decreasing the levodopa dose according to the individual sensitivity of the patient. An example of a multicenter clinical trial, in which the improper combination of levodopa with selegiline led to confusion and misinterpretation, is the one performed by the Parkinson's Disease Research Group of the United Kingdom (PDRG-UK) (Lees, 1995).

Quite unexpectedly, this group published an alarming paper claiming that parkinsonian patients treated with levodopa combined with selegiline show an increased mortality in comparison with the patients treated with levodopa alone (Lees, 1995). This finding was in striking contradiction to all other studies published in a variety of countries.

Shoulson summarized the results of the DATATOP study. Beginning in 1987, the study was conducted at 28 academic medical centers in the United States and Canada. After an average of 8,2 years of observation, the overall death rate of the subjects was 17,1% (137 of 800) or 2,1%/year. The final conclusion was that selegiline (10 mg/day) significantly decreased the time until enough disability developed to warrant the initiation of levodopa therapy. The effect was largely sustained during the overall 8,2 years of observation. *α-tocopherol produced no benefits!* The 2,1% per year mortality rate of the DATATOP cohort was remarkably low, about the same as an age-matched population without PD (Shoulson, 1998).

Birkmayer *et al.,* (1985) even found an increased life expectancy resulting from the addition of selegiline to levodopa treatment in PD. They compared in an open, uncontrolled study the long-term (9 years) effect of treatment with Madopar alone (N=377) or in combination with selegiline (N=564). The survival analysis revealed a significant increase in life expectancy in Madopar plus selegiline group.

The "idiosyncratic prescribing" (Dobbs *et al.,* 1996) of selegiline in combination with levodopa in the PDRG-UK study led to false conclusion by the authors. Comments uniformly pointed to the substantial overdosing of levodopa as the cause of the observed deaths with selegiline as an adjuvant in this trial (Dobbs *et al.,* 1996; Knoll, 1996; Olanow *et al.,* 1996).

Considering the peculiar pharmacological profile of selegiline, the unusual safety of this drug and the incurable nature of PD and AD, it is unfortunate that we are still in want of a multicenter, controlled clinical trial, designed to measure the prevalence of these neurodegenerative diseases in a cohort treated from at least age 60 with 1 mg selegiline daily.

It is worth mentioning regarding the potential neuroprotective effect of preventive selegiline medication against the manifestation of PD that according to a recent finding there is an inverse correlation between brain dopamine loss in PD and tissue norepinephrine levels (Tong *et al.*, 2006). Since selegiline, as a CAE substance, keeps the norepinephrine levels in the brain higher, this effect of preventive selegiline medication might be an additional factor that works against the manifestation of PD.

CHAPTER 7

Benefits of Selegiline in the Treatment of Alzheimer's Disease (AD)

In 1907 Alois Alzheimer first described the form of dementia that bears his name today. He was the first who pointed to a relationship between dementia and the extensive appearance of dense fiber-like tangles and darkly staining senile plaques in the cortical and hippocampal regions.

Based on the characteristic early symptoms and neuropathology of the disease, dementia cases are classified among four subtypes today:

Alzheimer's disease (AD) (50-75% of the cases). Early symptoms: Impaired memory, apathy and depression. Neuropathology: Dementia with cortical amyloid plaques and neurofibrillatory tangles.

Vascular dementia (20-30% of the cases). Early symptoms: Similar to AD, but memory less affected. Neuropathology: Cerebrovascular disease. Simple infarcts in cortical regions, or more diffuse multiinfarct disease.

Dementia with Lewy bodies (<5% of the cases). Early symptoms: Marked fluctuation in cognitive ability. Visual hallucinations. Parkinsonism. Neuropathology: Cortical Lewy bodies (α-synuclein).

Frontotemporal dementia (5-10% of the cases). Early symptoms: Personality and mood changes, disinhibition, and language difficulties. Neuropathology: Damage limited to frontal and temporal lobes.

AD is the major cause of disability in late-life. Only 2% to 10% of all dementia cases start before the age of 65 years. After this age the prevalence double of every five years. AD is conventionally diagnosed when cognitive decline affects a person's ability to carry out important routine activities.

The grave morphological changes lead to grave functional disturbances. For example, the loss of pyramidal neurons and their synapses leads to cholinergic and glutamatergic hypofunction. As the important role of these transmissions in cognitive and memory functions is well-known, the current symptomatic treatment of AD is based on correcting these hypofuntions. Acetylcholinesterase inhibitors (tacrine, donepezil, rivastigmine and galantamine) and memantine, a glutamate-modulating drug, are mostly used today to treat AD, but none of these drugs significantly modify the progress of the disease.

AD is the worst outward form of brain aging. An analysis of the prevalence of AD as a function of age makes it clear that this is just a grave form of the natural aging in the human brain. The mean age at the onset of AD is approximately 80 years, and the manifestation of the illness before the age of 60-65 years is very rare. In the age cohort 65-69, AD has a prevalence of only 1%. This increases to about 20% in the 85- to 89-year-old group and the risk of precipitating the disease can reach the 50% level among persons 95 year of age and over (Campion *et al.*, 1999; Hy *et al.*, 2000; Helmer *et al.*, 2001; Nussbaum & Ellis, 2003). The prevalence of PD over the age of 80 is only 1-3% (Tanner & Goldman, 1996).

In the population over 65, there is substantial sex (68% female, 32% male) and geographical (2.1% Japan, 5.2% Europe and 10% USA) differences in the incidence of AD (see Lockhart & Lestage, 2003, for review). By now the disease affects about 30 million persons world-wide. A sharp increase in the afflicted population is expected in the future, since the average lifespan is still increasing and the number of individuals over 65 is estimated to increase to 1.1 billion by 2050. It is, therefore, a pressing and no longer postponable necessity to find a safe and efficient preventive therapy to significantly decrease the prevalence of AD as soon as possible.

The ε4 allele of the apolipoprotein E (APOE) is the major risk factor for AD. The human APOE protein is a 299 amino acid glycoprotein which is expressed in several organs with the highest expression in the liver and brain. Prevailing evidence suggests that the differential effects of APOE isoforms on Aβ aggregation and clearance play the major role in AD pathogenesis. Since the APOE ε4 allele represents a loss of neuroprotective function, therapeutic strategies based on APOE propose to reduce the toxic effects of APOE 4 or to restore the physiological protective function of APOE (Kim *et al.*, 2009).

AD is characterized clinically by progressive cognitive impairment, impaired judgement, decision making and orientation, and leads finally to severe psychobehavioral disturbances and languague impairment. Due to the development of cortical amyloid plaques and neurofibrillatory tangles, AD is characterized by severe neuronal destruction, particularly in cholinergic neurons. Regarding the cause of AD the most popular hypothesis to date is that progressive cerebral accumulation of amyloid-β-protein [A$\beta_{(1-42)}$, Abeta protein] initiates a complex multicellular cascade that includes microgliosis, astrocytosis, neuritic dystrophy, neuronal dysfunction and loss, and synaptic insufficiency that results in neurotransmitter alterations leading to the impaired mnestic and cognitive functions. Since A$\beta_{(1-42)}$ is a neurotoxic agent, the hypothesis that this is a key molecule in the pathology of AD (Selkoe, 2000) is now widely accepted.

As neurotoxicity is thought to be inseparable from oxidative injuries, free radicals, calcium and inflammatory-mediated processes, agents with protective effect on cultured neurons, anti-oxidant compounds, and anti-inflammatory drugs are continuously tested in AD. For example: vitamin E and selegiline (Sano *et al.*, 1997; Birks *et al.*, 1999; Grundman, 2000; Thomas, 2000; Kitani *et al.*, 2002; Birks & Flicker, 2003), Ginkgo biloba extract (Ponto & Schultz, 2003), non-steroidal anti-inflammatory drugs (Etminan *et al.*, 2003), and estrogen (Schumacher *et al.*, 2003) are administered.

The first two studies demonstrating the beneficial effect of selegiline in AD were published in 1987 (Martini *et al.*, 1987; Tariot *et al.*, 1987). Series of clinical studies with small sample sizes confirmed thereafter the usefulness of this drug in the treatment of the disease (Agnoli *et al.*, 1990, 1992; Campi *et al.*, 1990; Falsaperla *et al.*, 1990; Loeb & Albano, 1990; Monteverde *et al.*, 1990; Piccinin *et al.*, 1990; Goad *et al.*, 1991; Mangoni *et al.*, 1991; Hardy & Lenisa 1992; Sunderland *et al.*, 1992; Burke *et al.*, 1993; Schneider *et al.*, 1993; Riekkinen *et al.*, 1994; Marin *et al.*, 1995; Lawlor *et al.*, 1997; Freedman *et al.*, 1998; Tariot *et al.*, 1998; Filip & Kolibas, 1999;).

The rationale and design of the first multicenter study of selegiline in the treatment of AD using novel clinical outcomes was published by Sano *et al.*, in 1996 and the results of this study were published a year later (Sano *et al.*, 1997).

The primary outcome involved the time that elapses until the occurrence of any of the following: death, institutionalization, loss of the ability to perform basic activities of daily living, or severe dementia. There were significant delays in the time taken for such primary outcomes to occur in patients treated with selegiline. The authors concluded that in patients with moderately severe impairment from AD, treatment with selegiline slows the progression of the disease.

Selegiline's value in the treatment of AD was reviewed. All unconfounded, double-blind, randomized controlled trials, reported before 31 December 1998, were the subject of a meta-analysis. Of the 27 trials taken into consideration, 14 met the inclusion criteria (Birks & Flicker, 2003; Birks *et al.*, 1999). Individual patient data were retrieved from eight trials on 821 patients. Summary data were extracted from five trials on 240 patients. For cognition there was a statistically significant difference between selegiline and placebo at 4-6 weeks and 8-17 weeks after randomization, but this disappeared at later assessments. There was a statistically significant difference at 4-6 weeks for activities of daily living, which disappeared at later assessments at 8-17 weeks (Wilcock *et al.*, 2002).

Beneficial effects of selegiline-treatment on cognitive dysfunctions of aged pet dogs and cats are in harmony with clinical experiences in AD. A decline in learning and memory can be demonstrated in dogs beginning as young as 7 years of age, but clinical cases of cognitive dysfunction syndrome (CDS) are seldom identified until 11 years or older. Pathological analysis of aged canine brains has documented the existence of Aβ plaques but no evidence of neurofibrillary tangles. Canines possess the identical amine sequence of Aβ found in humans. Based on neuropsychological, including reversal and spatial memory, testing and clinical trials, selegiline (Anipryl), dosed orally at 0.5-1.0 mg/kg daily, was the first agent approved for CDS therapy in dogs. Up to the present, the greatest amount of research on dogs has been conducted on selegiline studies (Milgram *et al.*, 1993; Ruehl *et al.*, 1995; Campbell *et al.*, 2001).

In experiments on canines 0.5 mg/kg (-)-deprenyl was administered orally. This is a low dose. Increased locomotor activity and stereotypes, including sniffing, have been noted in dogs at doses of 2 mg/kg and higher. Healthy young dogs trained in three tasks: 1) walking in a circle on commend, 2) retreating and sitting on a mat, and 3) acquiring and extinguishing an operant task (pawing a panel) learn faster following chronic oral treatment with 0.5 mg/kg (-)-deprenyl (Head & Milgram, 1992). Considering the pharmacological profile of (-)-deprenyl, it seems reasonable to conclude that the CAE effect was responsible for the observed beneficial behavioral effects of the drug.

Recent studies suggest that as many as 28% of pet cats aged 11-14 years develop behavioral changes which can also be described as CDS and this increases to 50% for cats of 15 years or older. Since selegiline showed in open trials a positive effect, the American Association of Feline Practitioners supports the use of a selegiline preparation (Selgian) for the treatment in CDS in cats.

None of the drugs used today change the hopelessness of patients who have already developed AD. It is in the center of our interest to find new possibilities modifying the progress of the disease. Research strategies in progress include: the search for antiamyloid agents targeting production, accumulation, clearance, or toxicity associated with $A\beta_{(1-42)}$ peptide, the metabolism of the amyloid precursor protein, vaccination or passive transfer of antibodies, the aggregation of $A\beta_{(1-42)}$ fragments produced by β- and γ-secretase, and last but not least, finding aromatic molecules for targeting Abeta-peptides. To review the disease-modifying treatment for AD see Galimberti and Scarpini (2011).

In a recent study, for example, the synthesis of selegiline-functionalized and fluorescent poly(allylcyano-acrilate) nanoparticles and their evaluation for targeting $A\beta_{(1-42)}$ peptide are reported. It was shown that the zeta potential value of the selegiline-functionalized nanoparticles dramatically decreased, thus emphasizing a significant modification in the surface charge of the nanoparticles. In comparison with the non-functionalized nanoparticles, there was no observed increase in the interaction between these selegiline-functionalized nanoparticles and monomeric form of the $A\beta_{(1-42)}$ peptide (Le Droumaguet *et al.*, 2011).

Since it is well known that dopamine modulates transmitter release at cholinergic and glutamatergic synapses in the hippocampus, it is self explanatory that enhancers of the dopaminergic transmission are beneficially influencing cholinergic and glutamatergic activities in the hippocampus. By itself the dopaminergic activity enhancer property would be, with all probability, enough for significant cognition improvement of selegiline in AD. Selegiline is traditionally administered in the dose which blocks MAO activity in the brain. Considering, however, the dose-effect-relation characteristic to the enhancer effect (Fig. **10**) it is obvious that nobody ever tried to investigate in patients the therapeutic effect of selegiline in the optimal low dose in which the drug exerts its specific enhancer effect.

(-)-BPAP is devoid of MAO-B inhibitory potency. As discussed in detail in Chapter 3 (-)-BPAP is today the most potent and selective enhancer of the catecholaminergic and serotonergic neurons in the brain stem. We demonstrated already in our first study on BPAP that the new compound significantly protected the cultured hippocampal neurons from the toxic effect of $A\beta_{(25-35)}$ fragment in the 10^{-13}-10^{-15}M concentration range and was in the higher (10^{-10}M) concentration ineffective (Knoll *et al.*, 1999, Fig 5).

Theoretically in the treatment of AD selegiline might be combined in the hope of a synergetic effect with the regular dose of a cholinesterase inhibitor. It is worth mentioning in this context that the co-administration of donepezil with selegiline, at doses that did not exert efficacy individually, significantly improved learning in mice pretreated with $A\beta_{(25-35)}$ fragment (Tsunekawa *et al.*, 2008). It is much to be regretted that this study is an example of those in which the authors administered subcutaneously superfluously high doses of (-)-deprenyl (1-3 mg/kg). In another study aged male rats were treated daily with rivastigmin (0.3 mg/kg), selegiline (0.25 mg/kg), and their combination for 36 days. The effect of this long term treatment was measured on cognitive performances (an object recognition test and a passive avoidance procedure). Both rivastigmine and selegiline improved significantly cognitive performances but the rivastigmine + selegiline combination was ineffective (Carageorgiou *et al.*, 2008).

AD and PD are incurable diseases. When diagnosed, the patients already passed recovery, since the neuropathological changes in the affected neurons are on an irreversible downward pass; they are driven to perdition. We have, in reality, no chance whatsoever to stop them on their mortal way. As discussed in Chapter 6, an   attempt,   however,   to   significantly   decrease   the   prevalence   of neurodegenerative diseases by slowing the natural aging of the threatened neurons *via* the preventive administration of a protective agent, such as selegiline, the only CAE substance in clinical use today, has a fair chance of success. It remains for future research to study the consequences of the preventive administration of BPAP the highly potent and selective synthetic enhancer substance which protected cultured rat hippocampal neurons from the deleterious effect of $A\beta_{(25-35)}$ fragment in as low as 10^{-14} and 10^{-15}M concentration (Knoll *et al.*, 1999).

Send Orders of Reprints at reprints@benthamscience.org

CHAPTER 8

Benefits of Selegiline in the Treatment of Major Depression Disease (MDD)

In 2010, World Health Organization made it public that depression affected 121 million people world-wide. There is still a continuous increase in the prevalence of MDD. The disease increased for example in the USA from 3.3% in 1992 to 7.0% in 2002 (Compton *et al.*, 2006). The most common time of onset of MDD is between ages 20 and 30 years. This is probably due to preexisting genetic vulnerability which is activated by stressful psychological and social conditions that catalyze the hypofunction of the catecholaminergic and serotonergic system in the brain stem.

MDD is characterized by the presence of a severely depressed mood that persists for at least two weeks. Episodes may be isolated or recurrent and are categorized as mild, moderate, or severe. Depression with episodes of markedly elevated mood (mania) is called bipolar disease, and the one without episodes of mania is called unipolar disease. Both the Diagnostic and Statistical Manual of Mental Disorders (DSM-IV-TR, American Psychiatric Association) and the International Statistical Classification of Diseases and Related Health Problems (ICD-10) have determined typical (main) depressive symptoms.

ICD-10 defines three typical symptoms: depressed mood, anhedonia (a psychological condition characterized by inability to experience pleasure in usually pleasurable acts), and reduced energy. Two of these disease symptoms determine the diagnosis of depression. DSM-IV-TR classifies depression as mood disorder and recognizes five subtypes of MDD.

Melancholic depression: Failure of reactivity to pleasurable stimuli, excessive weight loss, and excessive guilt.

Atypical depression: Mood reactivity (paradoxical anhedonia), significant weight gain (increased appetite), hypersomnia, leaden paralysis (sensation of heaviness in limbs), and social impairment.

Catatonic depression: Rare and severe form of MDD. The patient is almost stuporous.

Postpartum depression: 10-15% among new mothers. Can last as long as three months.

Seasonal affective disorder (SAD): Depressive episodes come in the autumn and winter, and resolve in spring. Diagnosed if at least two episodes have occurred in autumn or winter over at least a two-year period.

As discussed in Chapter 3, enhancer regulation in the catecholaminergic brain stem neurons play a key role in controlling the uphill period of life and the transition from adolescence to adulthood. The results of our longevity studies support the hypothesis that quality and duration of life rests upon the inborn efficiency of the catcholaminergic brain machinery, *i.e.* a high performing, long-living individual has a more active, more slowly deteriorating catecholaminergic system than its low performing, shorter living peer. Thus, a better brain engine allows for a better performance and a longer lifespan.

In contrast to PD and AD, today no firm correlation between morphological brain changes and the manifestation of MDD is known. Nevertheless, there is growing evidence for anatomical brain changes in depressed patients. Brain imaging studies found in MDD reduced volume of orbito-frontal cortex (Bremner *et al.*, 2002), and functional anatomical abnormalities in limbic and prefrontal cortical structure (Drevets, 2000). Glial loss and neuronal atrophy may contribute to these volume reductions, since according to experimental data glial loss in the prefrontal cortex induces depressive like behavior (Banasr & Duman, 2008).

Based on experimental and clinical data the current concept regarding the molecular neurobiology of depression is in harmony with the hypothesis that the catecholaminergic transmitters, norepinephrine and dopamine, and the serotonergic transmitter, serotonin, play a leading role in the manifestation of MDD, the mental disorder characterized by loss of interest in normal activities. Since the catecholaminergic system works as the engine of the brain, and its transmitters are responsible for alertness, attention, motivation, pleasure, and interest in life, it is obvious that whatever pathogenic biochemical lesion that leads to the hypofunction of the catecholaminergic machinery in the brain is a contribution to the manifestation of MDD.

There are a variety of symptoms of MDD: general emotional dejection, withdrawal and restlessness that interfere with daily functioning, such as loss of interest in usual activities; significant change in weight and/or appetite; insomnia; increased fatigue; feelings of guilt or worthlessness; slowed thinking or impaired concentration; and a suicide attempt or suicidal ideation, are all symptoms in harmony with the idea that a hypofunction of the catecholaminergic and serotonergic systems must be deeply involved in the manifestation of the disease.

On the other hand, the pharmacological spectrum of the most efficient drugs in the treatment of MDD, developed from the late 1960s up to the present, speaks in favor of the view that the development of a hypofunctional state of the catecholaminergic and/or serotonergic system is the concrete and final biological cause of the manifestation of MDD. This was immediately supported by the first breakthrough in the pharmacotherapy of MDD. It was discovered in the 1950s that iproniazid, a non-selective MAO inhibitor (Zeller *et al.*, 1952), increases the activity of the catecholaminergic and serotonergic neurons *via* the inhibition of the breakdown of their transmitters. It exerted a highly significant and characteristic psychostimulant effect in animal experiments and, as was first shown in 1957, was effective in the treatment of depression (Crane, 1956; Loomers *et al.*, 1957). MAO inhibitors fell, because of the "cheese effect", into disrepute, but new types of antidepressants were soon developed which further supported the monoamine hypothesis of depression (for reviewing the history see Ban, 2001).

In 1957, Kuhn reported that imipramine, a compound possessing multiple pharmacological effects, stimulates the noradrenergic and serotenergic neuronal activities in the brain and exerts a therapeutic effect in depressed patients (Kuhn, 1957). This finding was confirmed eight years later (Klerman & Cole, 1965), and followed by others such as Klein and Davis in 1969 and Angst in 1970. Further progress in the pharmacotherapy of MDD was the development of amitryptiline, the non-selective (prevailing norepinephrine) reuptake inhibitor, followed by the appearance of the selective norepinephrine reuptake inhibitors, such as desipramine and nortryptiline, and finally the selective serotonin reuptake inhibitors (SSRI), such as fluoxetine and flavoxamine were placed on the market.

Selegiline was the first MAO inhibitor to be free of the "cheese effect". The compound was originally developed with the intention to use it as a new spectrum antidepressant (Knoll *et al.*, 1965). Its antidepressant activity was first demonstrated by Varga (1965) and Varga & Tringer (1967) with the racemic form, and in 1971 with the (-) enantiomer (Tringer *et al.*, 1971). The first study that confirmed the beneficial antidepressant effect of (-)-deprenyl was published by Mann and Gershon (1980).

Once the beneficial effects of (-)-deprenyl were realized, first in PD and later in AD, the fact that it also had an antidepressant property remained unutilized. Even after especially interesting studies, its use for depression fell into oblivion. In a study performed by Birkmayer *et al.* (1984) on 102 outpatients and 53 inpatients, (-)-deprenyl was given together with (-)-phenylalanine, the precursor of PEA. (-)-Phenylalanin, in contrast to PEA, crosses the blood-brain barrier and after being metabolized in the brain, increases PEA concentrations. Nearly 70% of the patients achieved full remission. This outstanding clinical efficiency equaled electroconvulsive treatment without the latter's side effect, such as memory-loss.

Since (-)-deprenyl was primarily used in PD which is very often accompanied by depression, clinicians noticed the antidepressant effect of the drug (Youdim, 1980; Tom & Cummings, 1998; Miyoshi, 2001; Zesiewicz *et al.*, 1999). In a double blind evaluation Mendlewicz and Youdim (1983) found that (-)-deprenyl is a successful treatment in major depression. Some authors (Lees, 1991; Kuhn & Muller, 1996; Ritter & Alexander, 1997) found extremely high doses of (-)-deprenyl (40-60 mg/day) had marked antidepressant effect.

In 2002, Bodkin and Amsterdam published their first clinical trial with a new selegiline preparation, the selegiline transdermal system (STS). The STS was developed with the intention to deliver sustained selegiline blood concentrations sufficient to inhibit MAO-A and MAO-B in the brain, producing antidepressant effects without substantially inhibiting MAO-A in the gastrointestinal tract, thereby reducing the risk of hypertensive crisis. The Emsam patch is a matrix of three layers consisting of a backing, and adhesive drug layer, and a release liner that is placed against the skin. It is available in three sizes that deliver 6, 9, or 12 mg of selegiline per 24 hours. This was the first skin (transdermal) patch produced for use in treating MDD (Bodkin & Amsterdam, 2002).

Bodkin and Amsterdam performed a randomized, double-blind, placebo-controlled study that lasted for 6 weeks. The study enrolled adult outpatients with moderate-to-severe depression, all of whom met the DSM-IV criteria for MDD. The patients received either STS 6 mg/24 hr (N=89) or placebo (N=88) once daily. At the study's endpoint (6 weeks), the STS demonstrated significantly superior efficacy compared to placebo. Amsterdam confirmed the finding in a second study as well (Amsterdam, 2003). Based on these studies, STS (EMSAM) was approved by the FDA in February 2006 as the First Drug Patch for Depression.

It is remarkable that though we developed E-250 (later named (-)-deprenyl, selegiline), as a new antidepressant and the first clinical trial was performed on depressed patients in 1963, and the positive outcome of this trial was already mentioned as a personal communication in our first paper, published in Hungarian in 1964, and in English in 1965, and the antidepressant effect was thereafter confirmed in many papers, (-)-deprenyl was only 42 years later approved as an antidepressant, however, very luckily in the USA.

Animal studies have shown that the use of the 6 mg/24 hr patch can be administered without need for dietary restrictions (Gordon *et al.*, 1999; Wecker *et al.*, 2003). Azzaro *et al.* demonstrated that by using the 6 mg/24 hr selegiline transdermal patch, there is no need for dietary restrictions of tyramine in humans. They administered the oral tyramine pressor test to healthy males during treatment with the STS (6 mg/24 hr) in order to determine the risk of hypertensive crises. Following oral injection of dietary tyramine, they found that the patch is safe (Azzaro *et al.*, 2006). Patients receiving higher doses of Emsam (9 mg/24 hr and 12 mg/24 hr) need to follow dietary precautions. A further clinical trial confirmed that Emsam is effective in treating MDD and the 6 mg/24 hr patch can be used without dietary restrictions (Feiger *et al.*, 2006).

The 2001 expert consensus guidelines for treating MDD in geriatric patients recommended antidepressant treatment in combination with psychotherapy and stated that transdermal selegiline has shown promise in adult patients (Alexopoulos, 2011).

Atypical depression has characteristics inconsistent with melancholic depression (Matza *et al.*, 2003). Patients presented with nonmelancholic features include mood reactivity, hypersomnia, hyperphagia, and leaden paralysis, and they preferentially respond to MAO inhibitors. Quitkin *et al.* (1984) found selegiline effective against atypical depression. This open trial consisting of 17 patients made the finding questionable. However, McGrath *et al.* (1989) in a placebo-controlled trial proved the efficiency of selegiline in atypical depression. Patients unresponsive to 10 days of placebo were randomly assigned to selegiline (N=34) or placebo (N=64). The response rate in patients with atypical depression was 50% and 28% for selegiline and placebo, respectively ($P <0,05$). 12% and 22% of patients in the selegiline and placebo arms, respectively, discontinued the study. In article reviewing the history of approaches in treating depression with atypical features, the authors came to the conclusion that "…an introduction of the selegiline patch may improve outcomes for patients with atypical depression" (Stewart, 2007). In another paper, the authors came to the same conclusion: "…the transdermal formulation of selegiline may provide all of the efficacy of the older MAO inhibitors in treating atypical depression without causing as great of adverse events and no diet restrictions" (Rapaport & Thase, 2007).

The pharmacotherapy of depression is still inadequate. A recent meta-analysis of double-blind, randomized, controlled trials comparing antidepressants and placebo in adults with minor depression showed no statistically significant difference between antidepressents and placebo (Cipriani *et al.*, 2011). At present, even the clinically esteemed antidepressants are successful in a smaller percentage of patients with MDD. For example, according to a reliable study, only 1/3rd of the patients showed remission in response to a 12-week treatment with citalopram, a potent selective serotonin reuptake inhibitor (Trivedy *et al.*, 2006).

Nevertheless, there are case reports showing that some patients with severe MDD who failed to respond to reuptake inhibitors and other used treatments, found that selegiline can produce a prompt, dramatic therapeutic effect. For example, a 34-year-old man presented with severe refractory depression who had failed to respond to various antidepressants, augmentation therapy with lithium carbonate, and modified electroconvulsive therapy responded to selegiline (7.5 mg/day). This led to a complete remission of all depressive symptoms and reverted to his formal position at work after an interval of approximately 3 years (Higuchi *et al.*, 2005).

All in all, since the pharmacotherapy of MDD speaks in favor for the conclusion that hypofunction of the catecholaminergic and or serotonergic system in the brain is somehow closely related to the manifestation of the disease, the maintenance of these systems on a higher activity level *via* the preventive low-dose administration of selegiline and/or (-)-BPAP might also decrease the prevalence of MDD.

CHAPTER 9

The Unique Requirements for Preventive Medication to Slow Brain Aging

As briefly analyzed in Chapter 3 the enhanced activity of the catecholaminergic brain engine is responsible for full scale sexual maturity and is primarily responsible for the most delightful phase of life, the glorious uphill journey. Sexual hormones bring back the enhancer regulation in the catecholaminergic and the serotonergic neurons in the brain to the preweaning level, thus terminating developmental longevity. The postdevelopmental phase, the downhill period of life starts and lasts until the occurrence of "natural death". Since aging of the catecholaminergic system in the brain plays a leading role in the aging-related decay of physical and mental welfare, we need to start fighting against the aging of the catecholaminergic brain engine as soon as sexual maturity is reached.

The dopaminergic machinery is the most rapidly aging neuronal system in our brain. The dopamine content of the human caudate nucleus decreases steeply, at a rate of 13% per decade over age 45. We know that symptoms of PD appear if the dopamine content of the caudate sinks below 30% of the normal level. Experimental and clinical experiences show that daily dosages of (-)-deprenyl keeps the brain engine's activity on a higher activity level in humans. From sexual maturity, a low daily dose of selegiline (1 mg) is sufficient to significantly slow the pace of the aging-related decay of the dopaminergic neurons. "Even if we assume only a small protective effect of (-)-deprenyl in healthy humans against the age-related decrease in striatal dopamine, eg, from 13% per decade to 10% per decade, this translates to a minimum 15-year extension in average lifespan and a considerable increase of the human technical lifespan (TLS_h), which is now estimated to be 115 years" (see Fig. **6** in Knoll, 1992b).

As recapitulated in Chapter 5, we demonstrated in earlier longevity studies that male rats injected with (-)-deprenyl preserved their learning ability longer, lost their ability to ejaculate later, and lived longer than their placebo treated peers. In the opinion that the selective inhibition of B-type MAO in the brain is responsible for these beneficial effects, we performed our two longevity studies with 0.25

mg/kg (-)-deprenyl which blocks MAO B activity in the brain (Knoll, 1988; Knoll *et al.*, 1989; and Knoll *et al.*, 1994).

The discovery that (-)-deprenyl is a PEA-derived synthetic CAE-substance, and the development of (-)-BPAP, the tryptamine-derived, more potent synthetic CAE-substance than (-)-deprenyl, devoid of MAO-B inhibitory potency, drew our attention to this new subject. In May 2010 we started with Ildikó Miklya a still running longevity study which measures for the first time the effect of (-)-deprenyl and (-)-BPAP on the lifespan of rats on low doses of the enhancer substances. We started working with 2-month-old Wistar (Charles River) male rats. First we selected the proper CAE doses for the longevity study through shuttle box experiments.

In a modified version of the shuttle box (originally described by Bovet *et al.*, 1966) the acquisition of a two-way conditioned avoidance reflex (CAR) was analyzed during 5 consecutive days. The rat was put in a box divided inside into two parts by a barrier with a small gate in the middle, and the animal is trained to cross the barrier under the influence of a conditioned stimulus (CS, light flash). If it failed to respond within 5s, it was punished with a footshock (1mA), the unconditioned stimulus (US). If the rat failed to respond within 5s to the US, it was classified as an escape failure (EF). One trial consisted of 10s intertrial interval, followed by 20s CS. The last 5s of CS overlaped the 5s US. At each learning session, the number of CARs, EFs and intersignal reactions (IRs) are automatically counted and evaluated by multi-way ANOVA.

Tetrabenazine-treatment (1 mg/kg s.c.) depletes at least 90% of norepinephrine and dopamine from their stores in the nerve terminals of the catecholaminergic neurons in the brain stem. Due to the weak performance of the catecholaminergic brain engine, the activation of the cortical neurons remains below the level required for the acquisition of a CAR. The learning deficit caused by tetrabenazine-treatment can be antagonized by the administration of a synthetic CAE substance or an A-type MAO inhibitor, whereas selective inhibition of B-type MAO or inhibition of the reuptake of catecholamines and/or serotonin is ineffective (Knoll *et al.*, 1992a).

As was shown earlier (Fig. **10**), a bi-modal, bell-shaped concentration effect curve is characteristic to the enhancer effect. (-)-BPAP enhanced the activity of the noradrenergic neurons in the femto/picomolar concentration range ("specific enhancer effect"), and also in a 10 million times higher concentration range ("non-specific enhancer effect"). (-)-Deprenyl is a less potent CAE-substance than (-)-BPAP, but otherwise it exerts its specific and non-specific enhancer effect with the same characteristics as (-)-BPAP.

Fig. **18** shows that in this *in vivo* test too, a bi-modal, bell-shaped dose-effect-relation characterizes the enhancer effect of (-)-deprenyl. We selected for the longevity study two doses of (-)-deprenyl, 0.001 mg/kg and 0.1 mg/kg. The 0.001 mg/kg was selected as the optimal dose that exerted the specific enhancer effect. Regarding the dose with the non-specific enhancer effect, the less effective 0.1 mg/kg dose was selected for the longevity study because it allows B-type MAO to sufficiently oxidize the proper monoamines. The figure also shows that very high doses of (-)-deprenyl (5-10 mg/kg), due to the inhibition of MAO-A, are effective in antagonizing tetrabenazine-induced learning deficit.

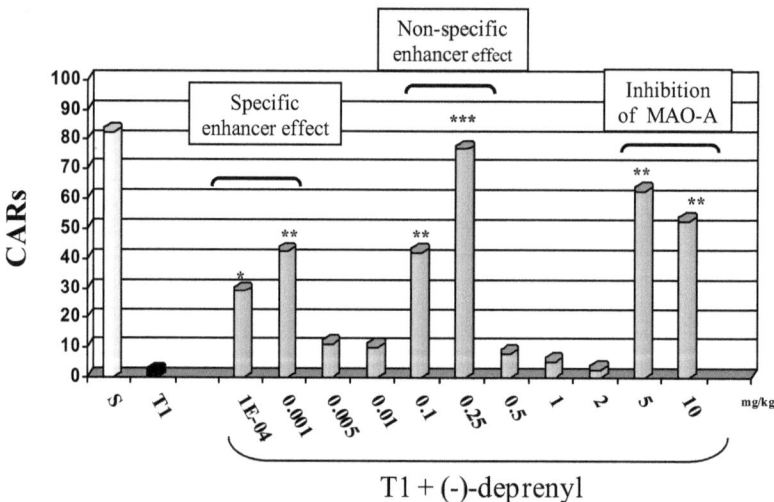

Figure 18: *Selection of optimal doses of (-)-deprenyl for the longevity study in the shuttle box.* Measured: (S) the ability of saline-treated (control) rats to fix conditioned avoidance responses (CARs); (T1) the inhibition of the learning ability of rats treated subcutaneously with 1 mg/kg tetrabenazine, one hour prior to training; [T1 + (-)-deprenyl] the ability of (-)-deprenyl to antagonize in a dose related manner the inhibitory effect of tetrabenazine.
Significance in the performance between the groups was evaluated by multi-factor analysis of variance (ANOVA). *$P<0.05$; **$P<0.01$, ***$P<0.001$.

Fig. **19** shows the dose-related effect of (-)-BPAP in the shuttle box. For the longevity study we selected the optimal dose that elicited the specific (0.0001 mg/kg) and the non-specific (0.05 mg/kg) enhancer effect. Since (-)-BPAP blocks the activity of MAO-A in higher than 2 mg/kg dose (Knoll *et al.*, 1999), it antagonized tetrabenazine-induced learning deficit in the extremely high dose-range (2-10 mg/kg).

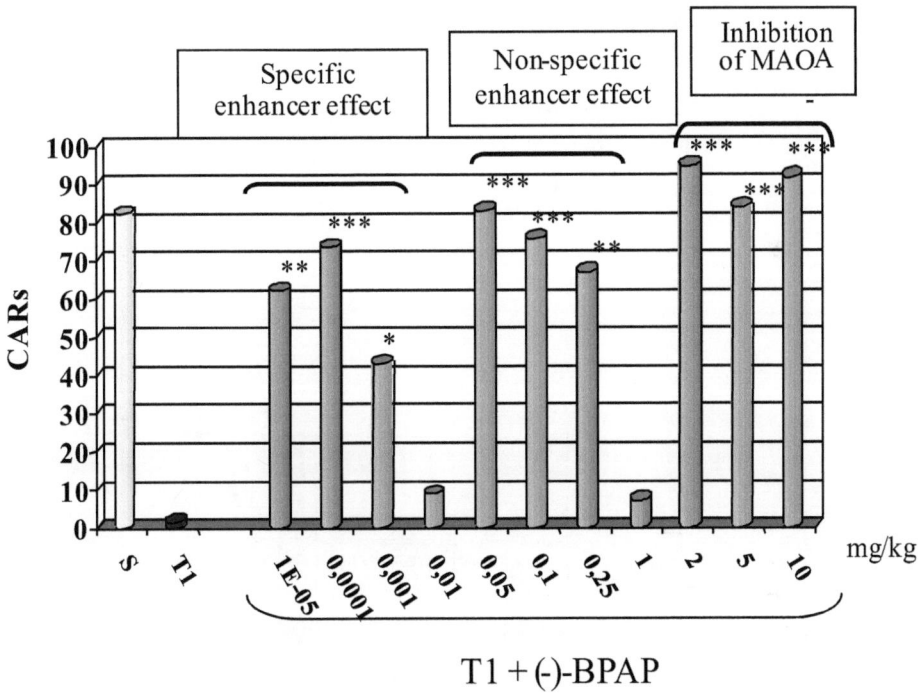

Figure 19: *Selection of optimal doses of (-)-BPAP for the longevity study in the shuttle box.* Measured: (S) the ability of saline-treated (control) rats to fix conditioned avoidance responses (CARs); (T1) the inhibition of the learning ability of rats treated subcutaneously with 1 mg/kg tetrabenazine, one hour prior to training; [T1 + (-)-BPAP] the ability of (-)-BPAP to antagonize in a dose related manner the inhibitory effect of tetrabenazine.
Significance in the performance between th.e groups was evaluated by multi-factor analysis of variance (ANOVA). *$P<0.01$; **$P<0.001$

Table **10** shows the course of our longevity study still in progress. As I write this Chapter, the rats have completed the 18th month of their life. Every three months we are testing the aging-related changes in their learning performance.

Table 10: Longevity Study on Wistar (Charles River) male rats. Treatment subcutaneously, 3 times a week (Monday, Wednesday, Friday).

Group	Treatment	Dose	Number of Animals
1	Saline	0.5 ml/kg	40
2	(-)-Deprenyl	0.1 mg/kg	40
3	(-)-Deprenyl	0.001 mg/kg	40
4	(-)-BPAP	0.05 mg/kg	40
5	(-)-BPAP	0.0001 mg/kg	40

Fig. **20** shows that, due primarily to normal aging of the catecholaminergic neuronal system in the brain stem, saline-treated 3-month-old rats are significantly better performing than their 1-year-old peers.

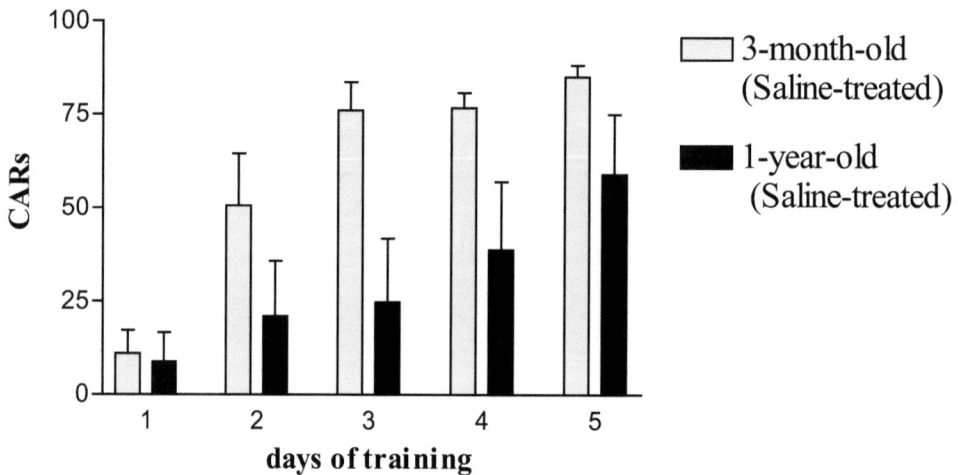

Figure 20: Experimental evidence that 3-month-old rats are significantly better learners than their 1-year-old peers *(P<0.001)*. Significance in the performance between the groups was evaluated by multi-factor analysis of variance (ANOVA). Rats were trained in the shuttle box with 100 trials per day. Conditioned avoidance responses (CARs).

On the other hand, Fig. **21** shows that due to the anti-aging effect of (-)-deprenyl, in the group of rats treated with 0.1 mg/kg (-)-deprenyl there is no sign of aging-related decay in the learning ability. This effect is in harmony with the results of our earlier longevity studies performed with the higher, MAO-B inhibiting dose of (-)-deprenyl (0.25 mg/kg).

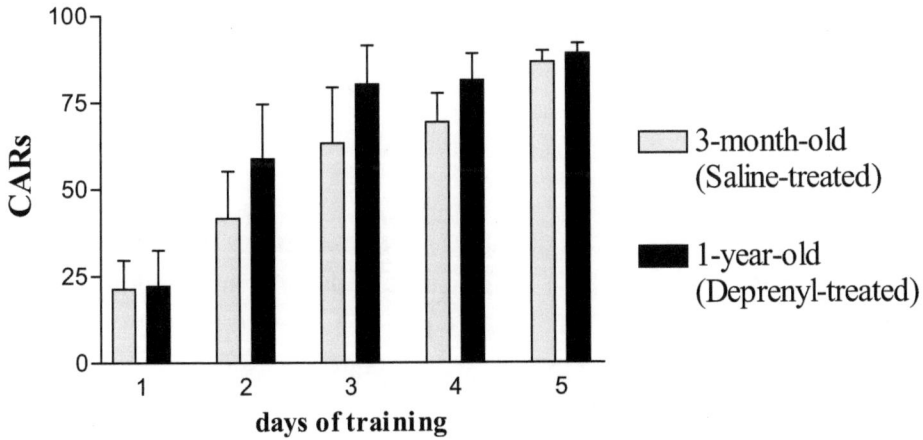

Figure 21: Experimental evidence shows that in rats treated with 0.1 mg/kg (-)-deprenyl there is no sign of aging-related decay in the learning ability. Rats were trained in the shuttle box with 100 trials per day. Significance in the performance between the groups was evaluated by multi-factor analysis of variance (ANOVA). There was no significant difference in the acquisition of conditioned avoidance responses (CARs) between the 3-month-old rats treated with saline and 1-year-old rats treated with (-)-deprenyl.

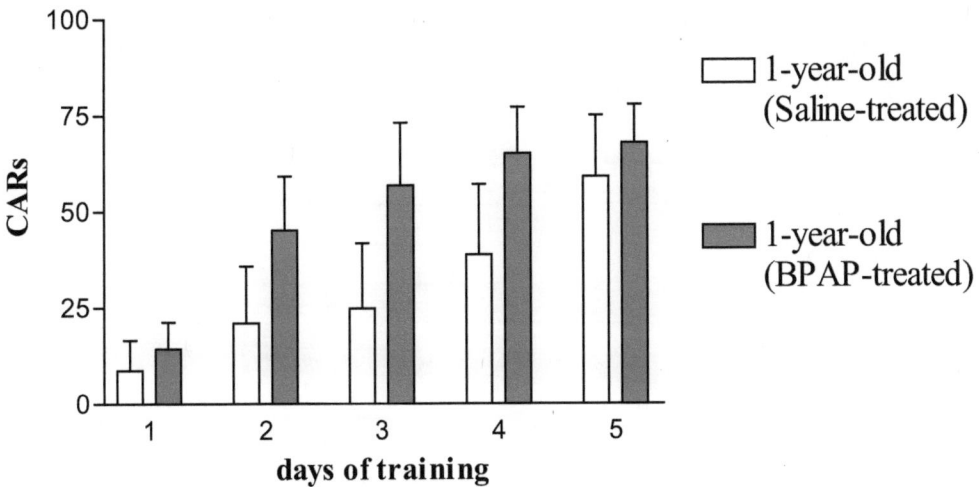

Figure 22: First evidence for the anti-aging effect of 0.0001 mg/kg (-)-BPAP. 1-year-old rats were treated for 10 months subcutaneously, 3-times a week, with the extremely low dose of (-)-BPAP (0.1 nanogram/kg) and their performance was compared to a group of rats treated similarly with saline. Rats were trained in the shuttle box with 100 trials per day. Significance in the performance between the groups was evaluated by multi-factor analysis of variance (ANOVA). The (-)-BPAP treated rats performed significantly better than their peers ($P<0.05$).

In the still running longevity study we already observed the effectiveness of (-)-BPAP. 1-year-old rats treated for 10 months subcutaneously, 3-times a week, with the extremely low dose of (-)-BPAP (0.1 nanogram/kg) performed in the shuttle box significantly better ($P<0.05$) than their peers treated similarly with saline (Fig. **22**).

Table **11** shows the number of rats deceased in various groups prior to the end of the 18th month of their life. It is already in this stage of the still running longevity study perceptible that treatment with 0.1 mg/kg (-)-deprenyl and 0.05 and 0.0001 mg/kg (-)-BPAP, respectively, slows the dying out of the rats.

Table 11: The dying out of Wistar male rats, prior to the end of the 18th month of their life, treated subcutaneously, 3 times a week, with saline and the enhancer drugs, respectively. Start of treatment at 2-month-age. In each group N=40.

Age (months)	Saline	(-)-Deprenyl 0.1 mg/kg	(-)-Deprenyl 0.001 mg/kg	(-)-BPAP 0.05 mg/kg	(-)-BPAP 0.0001 mg/kg
8th	1				
9th					
10th					
11th		1			
12th					
13th			1		
14th			2	1	
15th	3		1		
16th	1		1		1
17th	1	1	1	2	3
18th	3		1		1
Total number of deceased rats	9	2	7	3	5

As briefly demonstrated in Chapter 3, if we measure the amount of [^{3}H]-norepinephrine, [^{3}H]-dopamine or [^{3}H]-serotonin released from an isolated rat brain stem to electrical stimulation in a 3-min collection period and repeat the measurement in the presence of the optimal concentration of (-)-deprenyl or (-)-BPAP in which they exert their specific enhancer effect, the amount of the labeled transmitter released in response to stimulation is significantly higher. This is clear experimental evidence that a higher percentage of the enhancer sensitive neuronal population got excited under the influence of the synthetic enhancer substance. After a single washout, the neuronal population works immediately on the same level as before treatment with the enhancer substance (for review see Knoll 2001, 2003, 2005).

The fact that 0.0001 mg/kg (-)-BPAP is antagonizing tetrabenazine-induced learning deficit in the shuttle box is undeniably *primary in vivo evidence* for the unique mechanism through which the enhancer substances rev up the catecholaminergic brain engine. In optimally low doses of PEA and (-)-deprenyl, as well as, tryptamine and (-)-BPAP, there is an increase in the excitability of enhancer-sensitive neurons, thus we measured the enhancement of the impulse propagation mediated release of the transmitters from the catecholaminergic and the serotonergic neurons in the brain. In a proper low dose, (-)-deprenyl is a selective CAE-substance. (-)-BPAP, preferentially a serotonergic activity enhancer substance, is even as a CAE substance a much more potent enhancer than (-)-deprenyl.

Considering the preliminary results of the still running longevity study, demonstrated in Figs. **18-22** and Table **11**, there can be little doubt that the enhancer effect is responsible for the observed anti-aging effects of (-)-deprenyl and (-)-BPAP.

Using (-)-BPAP as the reference enhancer compound, we investigated on the isolated rat brain stem the effectiveness of all types of drugs used today to stimulate the activity of the catecholaminergic and/or serotonergic neurons in the brain (Miklya & Knoll, 2003). We found that in comparison to 50 ng/ml (-)-BPAP, 250 ng/ml desmethylimipramine, a norepinephrine reuptake inhibitor (Fig. 1 in Miklya & Knoll, 2003), 250 ng/ml clorgyline, the selective inhibitor of MAO-A; and 250 ng/ml lazabemide, the selective inhibitor of MAO-B (Fig. 3 in Miklya & Knoll, 2003), did not change the electrical stimulation induced release of [³H]-norepinephrine from the isolated rat's brain stem. Thus, they are devoid of an enhancer effect on the noradrenergic neurons in the brain stem.

We compared the enhancer effect of 50 ng/ml (-)-BPAP on the release of [³H]-dopamine from the rats' isolated brain stem with the effect of 50 ng/ml pergolide which stimulates both D_1 and D_2 dopamine receptors, and 50 ng/ml bromocriptine, which stimulates D_2 receptors (Fig. **5** in Miklya & Knoll, 2003). Neither pergolide, nor bromocriptine changed significantly the electrical stimulation induced release of [^{3}H]-dopamine from the isolated rat brain stem, thus they are devoid of an enhancer effect on the dopaminergic neurons as well.

Since (-)-BPAP preferentially enhanced the serotonergic neurons' activity, we measured the release of [^{3}H]-serotonin from the isolated rat brain stem in the presence of 10 ng/ml (-)-BPAP and compared this effect with the effect of 50 ng/ml fluoxetine, the selective serotonin reuptake inhibitor (Fig. **2** in Miklya & Knoll, 2003); and with MAO-A and MAO-B inhibitors, 250 ng/ml clorgyline and lazabemide, (Fig. **4** in Miklya & Knoll, 2003). None of these compounds enhanced the release of [^{3}H]-serotonin from the brain stem to electrical stimulation, showing that they are devoid of an enhancer effect on the serotonergic neurons.

The safety requirements for a preventive medication for life are obviously particular. A presently ignored, fundamentally important aspect therefore deserves special attention. Fig. **18** shows that (-)-deprenyl is antagonizing tetrabenazine-induced learning deficit in as low dose as 0.001 mg/kg. Fig. **19** shows that even an extremely low dose of (-)-BPAP, 0.00005 mg/kg, is more potent in this respect than 0.001 mg/kg (-)-deprenyl. The CAE substances, (-)-BPAP and selegiline, increase the activity of the catecholaminergic system **qualitatively** differently than any of the drugs used today for this purpose.

*What is the **qualitative** difference?*

Considering the outcome of our second longevity study with (-)-deprenyl, discussed in more detail in Chapter 2, the answer to this question is quite obvious. In this longevity study we picked out of a population of 1,600 rats the animals with the lowest and the highest sexual performance and demonstrated, on the one hand, that the high performing rats lived significantly longer than their low performing peers, and on the other hand, that regular dosages of (-)-deprenyl transformed the low performing rats into significantly higher performing ones, which lived then as long as their saline treated high performing peers (Knoll *et al.*,

1994). We assume that high performing, longer living rats possess a more efficient catecholaminergic brain machinery than their low performing peers and the treatment with (-)-deprenyl, a CAE substance, acts accordingly.

Since the natural enhancer substances, as well as their synthetic analogues increase the excitability of the enhancer sensitive neurons, the daily intake of (-)-deprenyl transforms the lower performing catecholaminergic neurons into higher performing ones. All in all, in the brain of the rats maintained on saline, the catecholaminergic system worked according to its natural abilities, whereas in their peers, maintained on (-)-deprenyl, the catecholaminergic engine worked better than its natural aptitude. Accordingly, we measured that with the passing of time, the (-)-deprenyl-treated rats, due to enhanced catecholaminergic activity, longer maintaining their ability to acquire a conditioned avoidance response in the shuttle box, were able to ejaculate longer. As a summation of the CAE effect with all the unmeasured beneficial effects, due to the enhanced activity of still unknown enhancer-sensitive brain mechanisms, the (-)-deprenyl-treated rats lived significantly longer than their saline-treated peers.

We observed the same changes in the activity of enhancer-sensitive cultured neurons if (-)-BPAP or (-)-deprenyl was present in the culture well. As discussed in Chapter 4, racemic BPAP, for example, inhibited β-amyloidal neurotoxicity in cultured hippocampal neurons in two distinct ranges of concentration, one with a peak at 10^{-13} M and one with a peak at 10^{-8} M (Fig. **5** in Knoll *et al.*, 1999). Whereas, in the normally working population only 20%, the high performing cells, survived in the presence of β-amyloid, the optimum concentration of BPAP (10^{-13} M) in the culture well made each neuron higher performing, and the surviving rate increased from 20% to 70%.

In a healthy human during the postdevelopmental phase of life taking 1 mg of selegiline daily, in which the drug acts as a selective CAE substance, the physiological milieu of the catecholaminergic neurons remains practically unchanged. The CAE substance transforms the lower performing enhancer-sensitive neurons to better performing ones. In striking contrast, all drugs used today harshly change the physiological milieu in the highly sophisticated living material *which is a quality of drug effect incompatible with lifelong preventive medication.*

(-)-Deprenyl-solutions for anti-aging medication (at present Dep-Pro™, 1 drop = 1 mg) are since the end of the last century in circulation. Thousands of notes on the internet give account of uncontrolled subjective experiences with selegiline, as an anti-aging compound. The overwhelming majority plays a great value on (-)-deprenyl, nevertheless it is obvious that from a scientific point of view this material is practically worthless.

Today, the average human lifespan is already exceeding 80 years in most highly developed countries. The longer we live the more compelling it is to slow the aging-related decay of physical and mental welfare. Since preventive anti-aging medication means treatment throughout postdevelopmental longevity, only the synthetic enhancer substances are receptive for this purpose. At present selegiline is the sole world-wide registered CAE substance. As a matter of fact, it is long overdue to produce *via* a proper trial on healthy volunteers, prima-facie evidence for the anti-aging effect of preventive selegiline medication. But let us hope all is not lost that is delayed. I am certain that the outcome of such a trial would open up new paths to improve the quality of life in the latter decades, which is very much on the map at present.

SUMMARY AND CONCLUSION

In light of the serious side effects of levodopa in PD, Birkmayer and Hornykiewicz tried in 1962 to achieve a levodopa-sparing effect with the concurrent administration of levodopa with an MAO inhibitor. Since combinations frequently elicited hypertensive attacks, they were compelled to terminate this line of clinical research.

In the early 1960s we succeeded in finding an exceptionally lucky structural modification of PEA and developed (-)-deprenyl/selegiline, the first selective inhibitor of B-type MAO. *In contrast to the known MAO inhibitors, it did not potentiate the effect of tyramine but inhibited it,* thus the compound was free of the "cheese effect". Considering this profile of (-)-deprenyl, Birkmayer *et al.* combined (-)-deprenyl with levodopa in PD and achieved the expected levodopa-sparing effect without signs of hypertensive reactions. Their study, published in Lancet in 1977, and the following Lancet Editorial in 1982, initiated the world-wide use of (-)-deprenyl in PD.

Today the most evaluated effect of the drug is its ability to slow the rate of the functional deterioration of the nigrostriatal dopaminergic neurones in patients with early, untreated PD, thus, to slow the progress of the disease. Using (-)-deprenyl in *de novo* parkinsonians was established in the DATATOP (Deprenyl And Tocopherol Antioxidant Therapy Of Parkinsonism) study in the USA and Canada, and was corroborated in important multicenter studies in France, Sweden, Finland, Norway and Denmark.

The DATATOP study authors thought that the formation of free radicals predispose patients to nigral degeneration and contribute to the emergence and progression of PD and expected that (-)-deprenyl, the MAO inhibitor, α-tocopherol, the antioxidant, and the combination of the two compounds will slow the clinical progression of the disease. They selected patients with early, untreated PD and measured the delay of the onset of disability necessitating levodopa therapy. The DATATOP study revealed that (-)-deprenyl, but not α-tocopherol, delayed the onset of disability associated with early, otherwise untreated PD. The discovery of the operation of a previously undetected enhancer regulation in the brain finally clarified the ineffectiveness of α-tocopherol in the DATATOP study.

The enhancer regulation is defined as: the existence of enhancer-sensitive neurons capable to change in a split second their excitability and work on a higher activity level, due to endogenous enhancer substances capable to enhance the impulse propagation generated release of the transmitter. PEA and its synthetic analogue, (-)-deprenyl, are specific experimental tools for studying the enhancer regulation in the catecholaminergic brain stem neurons. PEA is primarily a "catecholaminergic activity enhancer" (CAE) substance, but it is also a highly effective releaser of the catecholamines from their intraneuronal stores. This effect completely concealed the enhancer effect of this endogenous amine, which remained undetected. Amphetamine and methamphetamine, PEA derivatives with a long lasting effect, share with their parent compound the releasing property. (-)-Deprenyl was the first PEA/methamphetamine derivative that maintained the CAE effect of its parent compounds but completely lost the releasing property, thus enabling the discovery of the enhancer regulation in the catecholaminergic brain stem neurons. In the light of our present knowledge the CAE effect of (-)-deprenyl/selegiline seems to be primarily responsible for the majority of the beneficial therapeutic effects of the drug in PD, AD and MDD. α-Tocopherol, devoid of the CAE effect, remained ineffective in the DATATOP study.

On the one hand, (-)-deprenyl is a potent CAE substance. It increases the excitability of the catecholaminergic neurons in the brain stem. Thus the impulse propagation generated release of the transmitter is enhanced. (-)-Deprenyl exerts this effect at low, non MAO-B inhibiting doses. On the other hand, in higher doses which inhibit MAO-B activity selectively, (-)-deprenyl raises the brain concentration of PEA to enormous levels. PEA is the preferred substrate for MAO-B. Due to its continuous rapid breakdown by MAO-B, PEA has an extremely high turnover. In mammals treated with a dose of (-)-deprenyl which inhibits MAO-B activity completely, PEA levels increase by 1300 to 1500%. At a rate 5-10 times higher than the MAO-B inhibitory dose, (-)-deprenyl inhibits also MAO-A activity. To administer such high concentrations of (-)-deprenyl is contraindicated. (-)-Deprenyl, in a low dose range acts as a selective CAE substance and keeps the catecholaminergic system in the brain stem, the engine of the brain, on a significantly higher activity level.

From weaning until sexual maturity an increased enhancer regulation operates in the catecholaminergic and serotonergic neurons. This mechanism is responsible for the exuberant physical strength and mental vigor in the uphill period of life in mammals. Sex hormones bring back the enhanced enhancer regulation to the preweaning level. This mechanism terminates developmental longevity and constitutes the foundation of the transition from adolescence to adulthood.

The age-related decay in the supply of the brain with PEA, due to the progressive increase of MAO-B activity in the aging brain, and dopamine, due to the better than average decline of the dopaminergic neuronal activity during the postdevelopmental phase of life, are irresistible biochemical lesions of aging. The speed of deterioration of behavioral performances with the passing of time and longevity depends significantly on the pace of these lesions. (-)-Deprenyl, increases the supply of PEA and dopamine in the brain, which counteracts the aging process. Longevity studies have proven that male rats maintained on lifelong (-)-deprenyl preserved their learning ability longer, lost their ability to ejaculate later, and lived longer than their placebo-treated peers. The development of (-)-BPAP, a more potent synthetic enhancer substance than (-)-deprenyl, exerts its specific enhancer activity in femto/picomolar concentration.

It is easy to demonstrate that enhancer substances increase the excitability of enhancer-sensitive neurons. If we measure the amount of [3H]-norepinephrine, [3H]-dopamine or [3H]-serotonin released to electrical stimulation from an isolated rat brain stem in a 3-min collection period and repeat the measurement in the presence of the optimal concentration of (-)-deprenyl or (-)-BPAP, in which they exert their specific enhancer effect, the released amount of the labeled transmitter is significantly higher. This shows that the enhancer sensitive neuronal population, as a whole, works immediately on a higher activity level in the presence of the synthetic enhancer substance. After a single washout the neurons work immediately on their normal activity level again. Since neurons respond to stimulation in an "all or none" manner, it is obvious that only a part of the neuronal population (the most excitable ones) respond to the electrical stimulation. Since the enhancer substances increase the excitability of the neurons, in the presence of the enhancer substance a higher percentage of the neuronal population gets excited and the amount of the labeled transmitter released to the electrical stimulation is significantly increased.

Due to their CAE effect, selegiline and (-)-BPAP, maintain the activity of the catecholaminergic neuronal system on a higher activity level. None of the types of drugs used today to increase catecholaminergic and/or serotonergic neuronal activity in the brain share with selegiline or (-)-BPAP the enhancer effect. We tested clorgyline, the selective MAO-A inhibitor, lazabemide, a selective MAO-B inhibitor, fluoxetin, the selective serotonin reuptake inhibitor, pergolide and bromocriptine, the dopamine receptor antagonists. Between the CAE substances and the listed drugs it is the essential difference that selegiline and (-)-BPAP are synthetic analogues of physiological enhancer substances, and act accordingly. Whereas all types of drugs used today are harshly changing the physiological milieu of the neurons. Since we need to start our fight against the aging-related decay of physical and mental welfare as soon as sexual maturity is reached, and preventive medication is necessarily lasting through life, only enhancer substances are receptive to such treatment. In contrast to the drugs used today, they do not change the environmental milieu of the enhancer-sensitive neurons when administered in the specific enhancer dose-range. The enhancer substance is just changing the catecholaminergic neuron born with a lower excitability, to a better performing one. The results of our longevity studies are in harmony with this view. For example. In our second longevity study we selected out of a population of 1,600 male rats the 94 sexually lowest performing (LP) males and the 99 highest performing (HP) rats. We treated 44 LP rats with saline and 50 HP rats with (-)-deprenyl. The saline-treated LP rats lived 134.58±2.29 weeks, their (-)-deprenyl-treated peers lived 152.54±1.36 weeks, as long as the selected saline-treated HP rats (151.24±1.36 weeks). Thus maintenance on (-)-deprenyl transformed the low performing rats to high performing ones.

Experimental and clinical studies with (-)-deprenyl/selegiline strongly support the proposal that preventive administration of a synthetic enhancer substance during postdevelopmental life could significantly slow the unavoidable decay of behavioral performances with the passing of time, prolong life, and prevent or delay the onset of aging-related neurodegenerative diseases, such as PD and AD. *In humans, maintenance from sexual maturity on (-)-deprenyl (1 mg daily) is for the time being the only feasible treatment with a promising chance to reach this aim,* since selegiline is at present the only world-wide registered CAE substance.

Considering that the estimated number of individuals over 65 will reach by 2050 the 1.1 billion level, it is unfortunate that the implementation of a proper trial on healthy volunteers to measure exactly the anti-aging effect of Selegiline is since decades greatly needed.

EPILOGUE

Though "never marry your hypothesis" was and has remained my leitmotif, the outcome of our first longevity study fascinated me so greatly that I decided to undertake a self-experiment and started to take 1 mg (-)-deprenyl daily on January 1, 1989, at the age of 64.

Since February 1949, when I started working in the department, that I never left, my professional life remained essentially unchanged. I am still spending the whole day in the department and continue working at home far into the night.

To illustrate my present state of activity let me overview just the books I published since my 80th birthday on May 30, 2005.

In 2005, the monograph "The Brain and Its Self" (Springer) (176 pages) summarizing the essence of my lifework appeared.

In 2006, an extended version of my theory (266 pages) was edited in Hungarian by the Publishing House of the Hungarian Academy of Sciences.

In 2009, I wrote a book in Hungarian in which I tried to argue out my theory within the capacity of everybody. The book "Az emberiség jövője"(The future of mankind) (366 pages) was published in 2010, online, by the Semmelweis Publishing House in Budapest. I am planning to write next an English version of this book.

Now, as I am writing this eBook for Bentham Science, I have already completed my 86th year.

Nevertheless, what takes most of my time in the department is the still unchanged high-priority of research, since only in the continuous surveillance of running experiments roots the drainless resource of ideas.

All in all, after living 22 years on a never interrupted, low daily dose of (-)-deprenyl, I venture the remark that my self-experiment augurs so far well.

REFERENCES

Agnoli, A, Martucci, N, Fabbrini, G, *et al.* (1990), 'Monoamine oxidase and dementia: Treatment with an inhibitor of MAO-B activity', *Dementia,* 1:109-114.

Agnoli, A, Fabbrini, G, Fioravanti, M, *et al.* (1992), 'CBF and cognitive evaluation of Alzheimer type patients before and after IMAO-B treatment: a pilot study', *European Neuropsychopharmacology,* 2: 31-35.

Ahlskog, JE & Uitti, RJ (2010), 'Rasagiline, Parkinson neuroprotection, and delayed-start trials: still no satisfaction?', *Neurology,* 74: 1143-1148.

Alexopoulos, GS (2011), 'Pharmacotherapy for late-life depression', *The Journal of Clinical Psychiatry,* 72: e04.

Allain, H, Gougnard, J, Naukirek, HC (1991), 'Selegiline in *de novo* parkinsonian patients: the French selegiline multicenter trial (FSMP)', *Acta Neurologica Scandinavica,* 136:73-78.

Amsterdam, JD (2003), 'A double-blind, placebo-controlled trial of the safety and efficacy of selegiline transdermal system without dietary restrictions in patients with major depressive disorder', *The Journal of Clinical Psychiatry,* 64:208-214.

Angst, J (1970), 'Clinical aspects of imipramine' In: *Tofranil,* Stumpfli & Cie, Berne.

Archer, JR & Harrison, DE (1996), 'L-Deprenyl treatment in aged mice slightly increases life spans, and greatly reduces fecundity by aged males', *Journal Gerontology Series A – Biol Sci Med,* 51: B448-453.

Azzaro, AJ, Vanderberg, CM, Blob, LF, *et al.* (2006), 'Tyramine pressor sensitivity during treatment with the selegiline transdermal system 6 mg/24 h in healthy subjects', *Journal of Clinical Pharmacology,* 46: 933-944.

Bakhshalizadeh, S, Esmaeili, F, Houshmand, F, *et al.* (2011), 'Effects of selegiline, a monoamine oxidase B inhibitor, on differentiation of P19 embryonal carcinoma stem cells, into neuron-like cells', *In Vitro Cellular & Developmental Biology — Animal* 47:550-557

Ban, TA (2001), 'Pharmacotherapy of depression: a historical analysis', *Journal Neural Transmission,* 108:707-716.

Banasr, M & Duman, RS (2008), 'Glial loss in the prefrontal cortex is sufficient to induce depressive-like behaviors', *Biological Psychiatry,* 64: 863-870.

Bertler, A (1961), 'Occurence and localization of catecholamines in human brain', *Acta Physiologica Scandinavica,* 51:135-161.

Bickford, PC, Adams, SJ, Boyson, P, *et al.* (1997), 'Long-term treatment of male F344 rats with deprenyl: assessment of effects on longevity, behavior, and brain function', *Neurobiology of Aging,* 3:309-318.

Birkmayer, W & Hornykiewicz, O (1962), 'Der L-dioxyphenyl-alanin-effekt beim Parkinson syndrom des Menschen', *Archiv für Psychiatrie und Nervenkrankheiten,* 203:560-564.

Birkmayer, W, Riederer, P, Ambrozi, L *et al.* (1977), 'Implications of combined treatment with "Madopar" and L-Deprenil in Parkinson's disease', *The Lancet,* i:439-443.

Birkmayer, W, Riederer, P, Linauer, W, Knoll, J (1984), 'L-Deprenyl plus L-phenylalanine in the treatment of depression', *Journal Neural Transmission,* 59:81-87.

Birkmayer, W, Knoll, J, Riederer, P, *et al.* (1985), 'Increased life expectancy resulting from addition of L-deprenyl to Madopar treatment in Parkinson's disease: a longterm study', *Journal Neural Transmission,* 64:113-127.

Birks, J & Flicker, L (2003), 'Selegiline for Alzheimer's disease', *Cochrane Database System Review*, 1:CE000442.

Birks, J, Grimley, Evans J, Whitehead, A, *et al.* (1999), 'The efficacy of selegiline for the treatment of cognitive decline in patients with Alzheimer's disease: an individual patient data meta-analysis', *The University of Oxford, Department of Clinical Geratology.*

Blackwell, B (1963), 'Hypertensive crisis due to monoamine oxidase inhibitors', *The Lancet*, ii:849-851.

Blaschko, H, Richter, D, Schlossmann, H (1937), 'The inactivation of adrenaline', *Journal Physiology (London)*, 90: 1-19.

Bodkin, JA & Amsterdam, JK (2002), 'Transdermal selegiline in major depression: a double-blind, placebo-controlled, parallel-group study in outpatients', *American Journal of Psychiatry*, 159:1869-1875.

Borowsky, B, Adham, N, Jones, KA, *et al.* (2001), 'Trace amines: Identification of a family of mammalian G protein-coupled receptors', *Proceedings of the Natural Academy of Sciences USA*, 98: 8966-8971.

Boulton, AA, Juorio, AV, Downer, RGH (1988), *'Trace Amines: Comparative and Clinical Neurobiology (Experimental and Clinical Neuroscience)'*, Humana Press, Totowa, NJ.

Bovet, D, Bovet-Nitti, F, Oliverio, A (1966), 'Effects of nicotine on avoidance conditioning of inbred strains of mice', *Psychopharmacologia*, 10: 1-5.

Braga, CA, Follmer, C, Palhano, FL, *et al.* (2011), 'The anti-Parkinsonian drug selegiline delays the nucleation phase of α-synuclein aggregation leading to the formation of nontoxic species', *Journal Molecular Biology*, 405: 254-273.

Bremner, JD, Vythilingam, M, Vermetten, E, *et al.* (2002), 'Reduced volume of orbitofrontal cortex in major depression', *Biological Psychiatry*, 51: 273-279.

Bunzow, JR, Sonders, MS, Arttamangkul, S, *et al.* (2001), 'Amphetamine, 3,4-methylenedioxy-methamphetamine, lysergic acid diethylamide, and metabolites of the catecholamine neurotransmitters are agonists of a rat trace amine receptor', *Journal Molecular Biology*, 60:1181-1188.

Burke, WJ, Roccaforte, WH, Wengel, SP, *et al.* (1993), 'L-deprenyl in the treatment of mild dementia of the Alzheimer type: results of a 15-month trial', *Journal of the American Geriatrics Society*, 41: 1219-1225.

Campbell, S, Trettien, A, Kozan, B (2001), 'A noncomparative open-label study evaluating the effect of selegiline hydrochloride in a clinical setting', *Veterinary Therapeutics*, 2: 24-39.

Campi, N, Todeschini, GP, Scarzella, L (1990), 'Selegiline *versus* L-acetylcarnitine in the treatment of Alzheimer-type dementia', *Clinical Therapeutics*, 12:306-314.

Campion, D, Dumanchin, C, Hannequin, D, *et al.* (1999), 'Early-onset autosomal dominant Alzheimer disease: prevalence, genetic heterogeneity, and mutation spectrum', *American Journal of Human Genetics*, 65:664-670.

Carageorgiou, H, Sideris, AC, Messari, I, *et al.* (2008), 'The effects of rivastigmine plus selegiline on brain acetylcholinesterase, (Na^+, K^+)-, Mg^{2+}-ATPase activities, antioxidant status, and learning performance of aged rats', *Neuropsychiatric Disease and Treatment*, 4:687-699.

Carlsson, A (1979), 'The impact of catecholamine research on medical science and practice', In: Usdin E, Kopin IJ, Barchas J (Eds.), *Catecholamines: Basic and Clinical Frontiers*, Vol. 1, Pergamon Press, New York, pp 4-19.

Cipriani, A, Barbui, C, Butler, R, *et al.* (2011), 'Depression in adults: drug and physical treatments', *Clinical Evidence*, (online) pii:1003.

Cohen, G, Pasik, P, Cohen, B, *et al.* (1984), 'Pargyline and (-)deprenyl prevent the neurotoxicity of 1-methyl-4-phenyl-1,2,3,6-tetrahydropyridine (MPTP) in monkeys', *European Journal of Pharmacology*, 106:209-210.

Compton, WM, Conway, KP, Stinson, FS, *et al.* (2006), 'Changes in the prevalence of major depression and comorbid substance use disorders in the United States between 1991-1992 and 2001-2002', *American Journal of Psychiatry,* 163: 2141-2147.

Costa, E & Sandler, M (Eds) (1972), *'Monoamine oxidases – New vistas' (Adv Biochem Psychopharmacol 5)*, Raven Press, New York and North-Holland, Amsterdam.

Crane, GE (1956), 'Psychiatric side effects of iproniazid', *American Journal of Psychiatry,* 112:494-499.

Dalló, J & Köles, L (1996), 'Longevity treatment with (-)-deprenyl in female rats: effect on copulatory activity and lifespan', *Acta Physiologica Hungarica,* 84:277-278.

Davis, BA & Boulton, AA (1994), 'The trace amines and their acidic metabolites in depression an overview', *Progress in Neuro-Psychopharmacology and Biological Psychiatry,* 18:17-45.

Dobbs, SM, Dobbs, RJ, Charlett, A (1996), 'Multi-centre trials: U-turns by bandwagons and the patient left by the wayside', *British Journal of Clinical Pharmacology,* 42:143-145.

Drevets, WC (2000), 'Functional anatomical abnormalities in limbic and prefrontal cortical structures in major depression', *Progress in Brain Research*, 26: 413-431.

Dunn, S (Ed.) (1998), *'Dachau 29 April 1945. The Rainbow Liberation Memoires'*, Texas Tech University Press, Lubbock, Texas.

Ebadi, M, Sharma, S, Shavali S, *et al.* (2002), 'Neuroprotective actions of selegiline', *Journal of Neuroscience Research,* 67: 285-289.

Eckert, B, Gottfries, CG, Knorring L, *et al.* (1980), 'Brain and platelet monoamine oxidase in schizoprenics and cycloid psychotics', *Progress in Neuropsychopharmacology,* 4:57-68.

Elsworth, JD, Glover, V, Reynolds, GP, *et al.* (1978), 'Deprenyl administration in man; a selective monoamine oxidase B inhibitor without the "cheese effect"', *Psychopharmacology*, 57:33-38.

Esmaeili, F, Tiraihi, T, Movahedin, M, *et al.* (2006) 'Selegiline induces neuronal phenotype and neurotrophins expression in embryonic stem cells', *Rejuvenation Research,* 9:475-484

Etminan, M, Gill, S, Samii, A (2003), 'Effect of non-steroidal anti-inflammatory drugs on risk of Alzheimer's disease: systematic review and meta-analysis of observational studies', *British Medical Journal,* 327:128-131.

Falsaperla, A, Monici Preti, PA, Oliani, C (1990), 'Selegiline *versus* oxiracetam in patients with Alzheimer-type dementia', *Clinical Therapeutics*, 12:376-384.

Feiger, AD, Rickels, K, Rynn, MA, *et al.* (2006), 'Selegiline transdermal system for the treatment of major depressive disorder: an 8-week, double-blind, placebo-controlled, flexible-dose titration trial', *Journal of Clinical Psychiatry*, 67: 1354-1361.

Fischer, E, Heller, B, Miró, AH (1968), 'β-Phenylethylamine in human urine', *Arzneimittelforschung*, 18:1486.

Fischer, E, Spatz, H, Heller, B, *et al.* (1972), 'Phenethylamine content of human urine and rat brain, its alterations in pathological conditions and after drug administration', *Experientia*, 15:307-308.

Filip, V & Kolibas, E (1999), 'Selegiline in the treatment of Alzheimer's disease: a long-term randomized placebo-contoled trial. Czech and Slovak Senile Dementia of Alzheimer Type Study Group', *Journal of Psychiatry & Neuroscience,* 24: 234-243.

Fowler, CJ, Oreland, L, Marcusson, J, *et al.* (1980a), 'Titration of human brain monamine oxidase -A and -B by clorgyline and L-deprenyl', *Naunyn-Schmiedebergs Archiv für Pharmacology,* 311:263-272.

Fowler, CJ, Wiberg, A, Oreland, L, *et al.* (1980b), 'The effect of age on the activity and molecular properties of human brain monoamine oxidase', *Journal Neural Transmission,* 49:1-20.

Freedman, M, Rewilak, D, Xerri, T, *et al.* (1998), 'L-deprenyl in Alzheimer's disease. Cognitive and behavioral effects', *Neurology,* 50: 660-668.

Freisleben, HJ, Lehr, F, Fuchs, J (1994), 'Lifespan of immunosuppressed NMRI-mice is increased by (-)-deprenyl', *Journal Neural Transmission Suppl.,* 41: 231-236.

Galimberti, D & Scarpini, E (2011), 'Disease-modifying treatments for Alzheimer's disease', *Therapeutic Advances in Neurological Disorders,* 4:203-216.

Gibson, CJ (1987), 'Inhibition of MAO-B, but not MAO-A, blocks DSP-4 toxicity on central noradrenergic neurons', *European Journal of Pharmacology,* 141:135-136.

Goad, DL, Davis, CM, Fuselier, CC, *et al.* (1991), 'The use of selegiline in Alzheimer's patients with behavioral problems', *Journal of Clinical Psychiatry,* 2: 342-345.

Gordon, MN, Muller, CD, Shernman, KA, *et al.* (1999), 'Oral *versus* transdermal selegiline: antidepressant-like activity in rats', *Pharmacology, Biochemistry & Behavior,* 63: 501-506.

Greenshaw, AJ (1989), 'Functional interactions of 2-phenylethylamine and of tryptamine with brain catecholamines: implications for psychotherapeutic drug action', *Progress in Neuro-Psychopharmacology and Biological Psychiatry,* 13:431-443.

Grundman, M (2000), 'Vitamin E and Alzheimer disease: the basis for additional clinical trials', *American Journal of Clinical Nutrition,* 71:630s-636s.

Hall, DWR, Logan, BW, Parsons, GH (1969), 'Further studies on the inhibition of monoamine oxydase by MB 9302 (clorgyline)-I. Substrate specificity in various mammalians species', *Biochemical Pharmacology,* 18: 1447-1454.

Hardy, B & Lenisa, S (1992), 'Selegiline (L-deprenyl) – for Alzheimer's dementia', *On Continuing Practice,* 19: 5-10.

Hare, MLC (1928), 'Tyramine oxidase. I. A new enzyme system in liver', *Biochemical Journal,* 22: 968-979.

Hársing, RG, Magyar, K, Tekes, K, *et al.* (1979), 'Inhibition by (-)-deprenyl of dopamine uptake in rat striatum: A possible correlation between dopamine uptake and acetylcholine release inhibition', *Polish Journal of Pharmacology and Pharmacy,* 31:297-307.

Hauger, RL, Skolnick, P, Paul, SM (1982), 'Specific [^{3}H] beta-phenylethylamine binding sites in rat brain', *European Journal of Pharmacology,* 83:147-148.

Hayflick L (1985), 'Theories of biological aging', *Experimental Gerontology* 20:145-159.

Head, E & Milgram, NW (1992), 'Changes in spontaneous behavior in the dog following oral administration of L-deprenyl', *Pharmacology, Biochemistry & Behav,* 43: 749-757.

Heikkila, RE, Hess, A, Duvoisin, RC (1985), 'Dopaminergic neurotoxicity of 1-methyl-4-phenyl-1,2,5,6-tetrahydropyridin (MPTP) in the mouse: relationships between monoamine oxidase, MPTP metabolism and neurotoxicity', *Life Sciences,* 36: 231-236.

Heinonen, EH & Myllylä, V (1998), 'Safety of selegiline (deprenyl) in the treatment of Parkinson's disease', *Drug Safety,* 19: 11-22.

Helmer, C, Joly, P, Letenneur, L, *et al.* (2001), 'Mortality with dementia: results from a French prospective community-based cohort', *American Journal of Epidemiology* 154:642-648.

Higuchi, H, Kamata, M, Sudawara, Y, *et al.* (2005), 'Remarkable effect of selegiline (L-deprenyl), a selective monoamine oxidase type-B inhibitor, in a patient with severe refractory depression: a case report', *Clinical Neuropharmacology,* 28: 191-192.

Hy, LX, Keller, DM (2000), 'Prevalence of AD among whites: a summary by levels of severity', *Neurology,* 55:198-204.

Ingram, DK, Wiener, HL, Chachich, ME, *et al.* (1993), 'Chronic treatment of aged mice with L-deprenyl produces marked striatal MAO-B inhibition but no beneficial effects on survival, motorperformance, or nigral lipofuscin accumulation', *Neurobiology of Aging,* 14:431-440.

Janssen, PA, Leysen, JE, Megens, AA, *et al.* (1999), 'Does phenylethylamine act as an endogenous amphetamine in some patients?', *International Journal of Neuropsychopharmacology,* 2:229-240.

Johnston, JP (1968), 'Some observations upon a new inhibitor of monoamine oxidase in human brain', *Biochemical Pharmacology,* 17:1285-1297.

Jordens, RG, Berry, MD, Gillott, C, *et al.* (1999), 'Prolongation of life in an experimental model of aging in Drosophila Melanogaster', *Neurochemical Research,* 24:227-233.

Kaur, J, Sharma, D, Singh, R (2001), 'Acetyl-L-carnitine enhances Na+, K+-ATPase, glutathione-S-transferase and multiple unit activity and reduces lipid peroxidation and lipofuscin concentration in aged rat brain regions', *Neuroscience Letter,* 301: 1-4.

Kaur, J, Singh, S, Sharma, D, *et al.* (2003), 'Neurostimulatory and antioxidative effects of L-deprenyl in aged rat brain regions', *Biogerontology,* 4: 105-111.

Kelemen, K, Longo, WG, Knoll, J, Bovet, D (1961), 'The EEG arousal reaction in rats with extinguishable and non-extinguishable conditioned reflexes', *Electroencephalic Clinical Neurophysiology,* 13:745-751.

Kim, J, Basak, JM, Holtzman, DM (2009), 'The role of apolipoprotein E in Alzheimer's disease', *Neuron,* 13: 287-303.

Kitani, K, Kanai, S, Sato, Y, *et al.* (1993), 'Chronic treatment of (-)deprenyl prolongs the life span of male Fischer 344 rats. Further evidence', *Life Sciences,* 52:281-288.

Kitani, K, Minami, C, Isobe, K, *et al.* (2002), 'Why (-)deprenyl prolongs survival of experimental animals: Increase of anti-oxidant enzymes in brain and other body tissues as well as mobilization of various humoral factors may lead to systemic anti-aging effects', *Mechanisms of Ageing and Development,* 123:1087-1100.

Kitani, K, Kanai, S, Miyasaka, K, *et al.* (2005), 'Dose-dependency of life span prolongation of F344/DuCrj rats injected with (-)deprenyl', *Biogerontology,* 6:297-302.

Klein, DF & Davis, JM (1969), *'Diagnosis and drug treatment of psychiatric disorders'*, Williams & Wilkins, Baltimore.

Klerman, GL & Cole, JO (1965), 'Clinical pharmacology of imipramine and related antidepressant compounds', *Pharmacological Reviews,* 17: 107-141.

Knoll, B (1961), 'Certain aspects of the formation of temporary connections in comparative experiments on mice and rats', *Acta Physiologica Hungarica*, 20:265-275.

Knoll, B (1968), 'Comparative physiological and pharmacological analysis of the higher nervous function of mice and rats', PhD theses (in Hungarian), Hungarian Academy of Sciences, Budapest.

Knoll, J (1956), 'Experimental studies on the higher nervous activity of animals. V. The functional mechanism of the active conditioned reflex', *Acta Physiologica Hungarica,* 10:89-100.

Knoll, J (1957), 'Experimental studies on the higher nervous activity of animals. VI. Further studies on active reflexes', *Acta Physiologica Hungarica,* 12:65-92.

Knoll, J (1969), *'The theory of active reflexes. An analysis of some fundamental mechanisms of higher nervous activity'*, Publishing House of the Hungarian Academy of Sciences, Budapest, Hafner Publishing Company, New York.

Knoll, J (1976), 'Analysis of the pharmacological effects of selective monoamine oxidase inhibitors', In: GES Wolstenholme & J Knight (Eds), *Monoamine oxidase and its inhibition*, Ciba foundation Symposium 39 (new series), Elsevier, Amsterdam, pp131-161.

Knoll, J (1978), 'The possible mechanism of action of (-)deprenyl in Parkinson's disease', *Journal Neural Transmission,* 43:177-198.

Knoll, J (1981a), 'Can the suicide inactivation of MAO by deprenyl explain its pharmacological effects?', In: TP Singer & N Ondarza (Eds), *Molecular Basis of Drug Action*, Elsevier, Amsterdam, pp185-201.

Knoll, J (1981b), 'The pharmacology of selective MAO inhibitors', In: MBH Youdim & ES Paykel (Eds), *Monoamine oxidase inhibitors-the state of the art,* John Wiley and Sons Ltd, London, pp 45-61.

Knoll, J (1981c), 'Further experimental support to the concept that (-)deprenyl facilitates dopaminergic neurotransmissionin the brain', In: K Kamijo, E Usdin, T Nagatsu (Eds), *Monoamine Oxidase. Basic and Clinical Frontiers*, Excerpta Medica, Amsterdam, pp 230-240.

Knoll, J (1982), 'Selective inhibition of B type monoamine oxidase in the brain: a drug strategy to improve the quality of life in senescence', In: JA Keverling Buisman (Ed), *Strategy in drug research*, Elsevier, Amsterdam, pp 107-135.

Knoll, J (1983), 'Deprenyl (selegiline). The history of its development and pharmacological action', *Acta Neurologica Scandinavica Suppl,* 95:57-80.

Knoll, J (1985), 'The facilitation of dopaminergic activity in the aged brain by (-)deprenyl. A proposal for a strategy to improve the quality of life in senescence', *Mechanisms of Ageing and Development,* 30:109-122.

Knoll, J (1986a), 'Striatal dopamine, aging and deprenyl', In: J Borsy, L Kerecsen, L György (Eds), *Dopamine, ageing and diseases*, Pergamon Press, Akadémiai Kiadó (Publishing House of the Hungarian Academy of Sciences), Budapest, pp 7-26.

Knoll, J (1986b), 'The pharmacology of (-)deprenyl', *Journal Neural Transmission Suppl,* 22:75-89.

Knoll, J (1986c), 'Role of B-type monoamine oxidase inhibition in the treatment of Parkinson's disease. An update', In: NS Shah, AG Donald (Eds), *Movement disorders*, Plenum Press, New York, pp 53-81.

Knoll, J (1987), 'R-(-)Deprenyl (Selegiline, Movergan[R]) facilitates the activity of the nigrostriatal dopaminergic neuron', *Journal Neural Transmission,* 25:45-66.

Knoll, J (1988), 'The striatal dopamine dependency of lifespan in male rats. Longevity study with (-)deprenyl', *Mechanisms of Ageing and Development,* 46:237-262.

Knoll, J (1989), 'The pharmacology of selegiline /(-)deprenyl/', *Acta Neurologica Scandinavica,* 126:83-91.

Knoll, J (1990), 'Nigrostriatal dopaminergic activity, deprenyl treatment, and longevity', *Advances in Neurology,* 53:425-429.

Knoll, J (1992a), 'Pharmacological basis of the therapeutic effect of (-)deprenyl in age-related neurological diseases', *Medicinal Research Reviews,* 12:505-524.

Knoll, J (1992b), '(-)Deprenyl-medication: A strategy to modulate the age-related decline of the striatal dopaminergic system', *Journal of the American Geriatrics Society,* 40:839-847.

Knoll, J (1993a), 'The pharmacological basis of the beneficial effect of (-)deprenyl (selegiline) in Parkinson's and Alzheimer's diseases', *Journal Neural Transmission Suppl,* 40:69-91.

Knoll, J (1993b), 'The pharmacological basis of the therapeutic effect of (-)-deprenyl in age-related neurological diseases', In: I Szelenyi (Ed), *Inhibitors of monoamine oxidase B. Pharmacology and clinical use in neurodegenerative disorders*, Birkhäuser Verlag, Basel, pp 145-168.

Knoll, J (1993c), 'Some clinical implication of MAO-B inhibition', In: H Yasuhara, SH Parvez, K Oguchi, M Sandler, T Nagatsu (Eds), *Monoamine oxidase: basic and clinical aspects*, VSP Utrecht, The Netherlands, pp 197-217.

Knoll, J (1994), 'Memories of my 45 years in research', *Pharmacology & Toxicology,* 75:65-72.

Knoll, J (1995), 'Rationale for (-)deprenyl (selegiline) medication in Parkinson's disease and in prevention of age-related nigral changes', *Biomedicine & Pharmacotherapy*, 49:187-195.

Knoll, J (1996), '(-)Deprenyl (selegiline) in Parkinson's disease: a pharmacologist's comment', *Biomedicine & Pharmacotherapy,* 50:315-317.

Knoll, J (1998), '(-)Deprenyl (selegiline) a catecholaminergic activity enhancer (CAE) substance acting in the brain', *Pharmacology & Toxicology,* 82:57-66.

Knoll, J (2001), 'Antiaging compounds: (-)Deprenyl (Selegiline) and (-)1-(benzofuran-2-yl)-2-propylaminopentane, (-)BPAP, a selective highly potent enhancer of the impulse propagation mediated release of catecholamines and serotonin in the brain', *CNS Drug Reviews*, 7:317-345.

Knoll, J (2003), 'Enhancer regulation/endogenous and synthetic enhancer compounds: A neurochemical concept of the innate and acquired drives', *Neurochemical Research,* 28:1187-1209.

Knoll, J (2005), *'The brain and its self. A neurochemical concept of the innate and acquired drives'*, Springer, Berlin, Heidelberg, New York.

Knoll, J & Magyar, K (1972), 'Some puzzling effects of monoamine oxidase inhibitors', *Advances in Biochemical Psychopharmacology,* 5:393-408.

Knoll, J & Miklya, I (1994), 'Multiple, small dose administration of (-)deprenyl enhances catecholaminergic activity and diminishes serotoninergic activity in the brain and these effects are unrelated to MAO-B inhibition', *Archives internationales de Pharmacodynamie et de Thérapie*, 328:1-15.

Knoll, J & Miklya, I (1995), 'Enhanced catecholaminergic and serotoninergic activity in rat brain from weaning to sexual maturity. Rationale for prophylactic (-)deprenyl (selegiline) medication', *Life Sciences,* 56:611-620.

Knoll, J, Kelemen, K, Knoll, B (1955a), 'Experimental studies on the higher nervous activity of animals. I. A method for the elaboration of a non-extinguishable conditioned reflex in the rat', *Acta Physiologica Hungarica,* 8:327-345.

Knoll, J, Kelemen, K, Knoll, B (1955b), 'Experimental studies on the higher nervous activity of animals. II. Differences in the state of function of the cells constituting the cortical representation of the unconditioned reflex in extinguishable and non-extinguishable conditioned reflexes', *Acta Physiologica Hungarica,* 8:347-367.

Knoll, J, Kelemen, K, Knoll, B (1955c), 'Experimental studies on the higher nervous activity of animals. III. Experimental studies on the active conditioned reflex', *Acta Physiologica Hungarica,* 8:369-388.

Knoll, J, Kelemen, K, Knoll, B (1956), 'Experimental studies on the higher nervous activity of animals. IV. A method for elaborating and studying an active conditioned feeding reflex. Experimental analysis of differences between active conditioned defensive and feeding reflexes', *Acta Physiologica Hungarica,* 9:99-109.

Knoll, J, Ecsery, Z, Kelemen, K, Nievel, J, Knoll, B (1964), 'Phenylisopropylmethyl-propinylamine HCL (E-250) egy új hatásspektrumú pszichoenergetikum', *MTA V. Oszt. Közl.* 15: 231-238 (in Hungarian).

Knoll, J, Ecseri, Z, Kelemen, K, Nievel, J, Knoll, B (1965), 'Phenylisopropylmethyl propinylamine (E-250) a new psychic energizer', *Archives internationales de Pharmacodynamie et de Thérapie,* 155:154-164.

Knoll, J, Vizi, ES, Somogyi, G (1968), 'Phenylisopropylmethylpropinylamine (E-250), a monoamine oxidase inhibitor antagonizing the effects of tyramine', *Arzneimittelforschung* 18:109-112.

Knoll, J, Yen, TT, Dalló, J (1983), 'Long-lasting, true aphrodisiac effect of (-)deprenyl in sexually sluggish old male rats', *Modern Problems in Pharmacopsychiatry,* 19:135-153.

Knoll, J, Dalló, J, Yen, TT (1989), 'Striatal dopamine, sexual activity and lifespan. Longevity of rats treated with (-)deprenyl', *Life Sciences,* 45:525-531.

Knoll, J, Knoll, B, Török, Z, *et al.* (1992a), 'The pharmacology of 1-phenyl-2-propylaminopentane (PPAP), a deprenyl-derived new spectrum psychostimulant', *Archives internationales de Pharmacodynamie et de Thérapie,* 316:5-29.

Knoll, J, Tóth, V, Kummert, M, Sugár, J (1992b), '(-)Deprenyl and (-)parafluorodeprenyl-treatment prevents age-related pigment changes in the substantia nigra. A TV-image analysis of neuromelanin', *Mechanisms of Ageing and Develoopment,* 63:157-163.

Knoll, J, Yen, TT, Miklya, I (1994), 'Sexually low performing male rats die earlier than their high performing peers and (-)deprenyl treatment eliminates this difference', *Life Sciences* 54:1047-1057.

Knoll, J, Miklya, I, Knoll, B, Markó, R, Kelemen, K (1996a), '(-)Deprenyl and (-)1-phenyl-2-propylaminopentane, [(-)PPAP], act primarily as potent stimulants of action potential-transmitter release coupling in the catecholaminergic neurons', *Life Sciences,* 58: 817-827.

Knoll, J, Knoll, B, Miklya, I (1996b), 'High performing rats are more sensitive toward catecholaminergic activity enhancer (CAE) compounds than their low performing peers', *Life Sciences,* 58:945-952.

Knoll, J, Miklya, I, Knoll, B, Markó, R, Rácz, D (1996c), 'Phenylethylamine and tyramine are mixed-acting sympathomimetic amines in the brain', *Life Sciences,* 58:2101-2114.

Knoll, J, Yoneda, F, Knoll, B, Ohde, H, Miklya, I (1999), '(-)l-(Benzofuran-2-yl)-2-propylaminopentane, [(-)BPAP], a selective enhancer of the impulse propagation mediated release of catecholamines and serotonin in the brain', *British Journal of Pharmacology,* 128:1723-1732.

Knoll, J, Miklya, I, Knoll, B, Dalló, J (2000), 'Sexual hormones terminate in the rat the significantly enhanced catecholaminergic/serotoninergic tone in the brain characteristic to the post-weaning period', *Life Sciences,* 67:765-773.

Knoll, J, Miklya, I, Knoll, B (2002), 'Stimulation of the catecholaminergic and serotoninergic neurons in the rat brain by R-(-)-1-(benzofuran-2-yl)-2-propylaminopentane, (-)-BPAP', *Life Sciences,* 71:2137-2144.

Kuhn, R (1957), 'Über die Behandlung depressiver Zustände mit einem Imonodibenzilderivat', *Schweitzer Medizinische Wochenschrift,* 36:1135-1139.

Kuhn, W & Muller, T (1996), 'The clinical potential of deprenyl in neurological and psychiatric disorders', *Journal Neural Transmission Suppl,* 48:85-93.

Lancet Editorial (1982), 'Deprenyl in Parkinson's Disease', *The Lancet* Vol.2, No.8300, (September 25) pp. 695-696.

Langston, JW & Ballard, PA Jr. (1983), 'Parkinson's disease in a chemist working with 1-methyl-4-phenyl-1,2,5,6-tetrahydropyridine', *New England Journal of Medicine,* 309: 310.

Langston, JW, Ballard, P, Tetrud, JW, *et al.* (1983), 'Chronic Parkinsonism in humans due to a product of meperidine analog synthesis', *Science,* 219: 979-980.

Langston, JW, Forno, LS, Rebert, CS, *et al.* (1984), 'Selective nigral toxicity after systemic administration of 1-methyl-4-phenyl-1,2,5,6-tetrahydropyridine (MPTP) in the squirrel monkey', *Brain Research,* 292: 390-394.

Larsen, JP, Boas, J, Erdal, JE (1999), 'Does selegiline modify the progression of early Parkinson's disease? Results from a five-year study', The Norwegian-Danish Study Group. *European Journal of Neurology,* 6:539-547.

Lawlor, BA, Aisen, PS, Green, C, *et al.* (1997), 'Selegiline in the treatment of behaviour disturbance in Alzheimer's disease', *International Journal of Geriatric Psychiatry,* 12: 319-322.

Lindemann, L, Ebeling, M, Krotochwil, NA, *et al.* (2005), 'Trace amine-associated receptors from structurally and functionally distinct subfamilies of novel G protein-coupled receptors', *Genomics,* 85: 372-385.

Le Droumaguet, B, Souguir, H, Brambilla, D, *et al.* (2011), 'Selegiline-functionalized, PEGylated poly(alkylcyanoacrylate)nanoparticles: investigation of interaction with amyloid-β peptide and surface reorganization', *International Journal of Pharmaceutics* 416: 453-460.

Lees, AJ (1991), 'Selegiline hydrochloride and cognition', *Acta Neurologica Scandinavica Suppl,* 136:91-94.

Lees, AJ (1995), 'Comparison of therapeutic effects and mortality data of levodopa and levodopa combined with selegiline in patients with early, mild Parkinson's disease', *British Medical Journal,* 311:1602-1607.

Lockhart, BP & Lestage, PJ (2003), 'Cognition enhancing or neuroprotective compounds for the treatment of cognitive disorders: why? when? which?', *Experimental Gerontology,* 38:119-128.

Loeb, C & Albano, C (1990), 'Selegiline – A new approach to DAT treatment', *European Conference on Parkinson's Disease and Extrapiramidal Disorders.* Rome, July 10-14.

Loomers, HP, Saunders, JC, Kline, NS (1957), 'A clinical and pharmacodynamic evaluation of iproniazid as a psychic energizer', *Psychiatric Research Report,* 8:129-141.

Magyar, K, Vizi, ES, Ecseri, Z, Knoll, J (1967) 'Comparative pharmacological analysis of the optical isomers of phenyl-isopropyl-methyl-propinylamine (E-250)', *Acta Physiol Hung* 32:377-387.

Mangoni, A, Grassi, MP, Frattola, L, *et al.* (1991), 'Effects of a MAO-B inhibitor in the treatment of Alzheimer disease', *European Neurology,* 31:100-107.

Mann, JJ & Gershon, S (1980), 'A selective monoamine oxidase-B inhibitor in endogenous depression', *Life Sciences,* 26:877-882.

Mantle, TJ, Garrett, NJ, Tipton, KF (1976), 'The development of monoamine oxidase in rat liver and brain', *FEBS Letters,* 64:227-230.

Marin, DB, Bierer, LM, Lawlor, BA, *et al.* (1995), 'L-Deprenyl and physostigmin for the treatment of Alzheimer's disease', *Psychiatric Research,* 58: 181-189.

Markey, SP, Johannessen, JN, Chiueh, CC, *et al.* (1984), 'Intraneuronal generation of a pyridinium metabolite may cause drug-induced parkinsonism', *Nature,* 311: 464-467.

Martin, C (1977), 'Sexual activity in the aging male', In: J Money, H Musaph (Eds), *Handbook of sexology,* Elsevier, Amsterdam, pp. 813-824.

Martini, E, Pataky, I, Szilágyi, K, *et al.* (1987), 'Brief information on an early phase-II study with (-)deprenyl in demented patients', *Pharmacopsychiatry,* 20:256-257.

Matza, LS, Revicki, DA, Davidson, JR, *et al.* (2003), 'Depression with atypical features in the National Comorbidity Survey: classification, description, and consequences', *Archives of General Psychiatry,* 60: 817-826.

McGeer, EG, McGeer, PL, Wada, JK (1971), 'Distribution of tyrosine hydroxylase in human and animal brain', *Journal of Neurochemistry,* 18:1647-1658.

McGrath, PJ, Steward, JW, Harrison, W, *et al.* (1989), 'A placebo-controlled trial of L-deprenyl in atypical depression', *Pschopharmacology Bulletin,* 25:63-67.

Mehta, SH, Morgan, JC, Sethi, KD (2010), 'Does rasagiline have a disease-modifying effect on Parkinson's disease?', *Current Neurology and Neuroscience Reports*, 10: 413-416.

Mendlewicz, J & Youdim, MB (1983), 'L-Deprenil, a selective monoamine oxidase type B inhibitor, in the treatment of depression: a double blind evaluation', *British Journal of Pschiatry*, 142:508-511.

Miklya, I (2011), 'The Knoll-Concept to Decrease the Prevalence of Parkinson's Disease', Chapter 5 In: DI Finkelstein (Ed), *Towards new therapies for Parkinson's Disease,* InTech, pp. 77-100.

Miklya, I & Knoll, J (2003), 'Analysis of the effect of (-)-BPAP, a selective enhancer of the impulse propagation mediated release of catecholamines and serotonin in the brain', *Life Sciences,* 72:2915-2921.

Miklya, I, Knoll, B, Knoll, J (2003), 'A pharmacological analysis elucidating why, in contrast to (-)-deprenyl (selegiline) α-tocopherol was ineffective in the DATATOP study', *Life Sciences.* 72:2641-2648.

Milgram, MW, Racine, RJ, Nellis, P, *et al.* (1990), 'Maintenance on L-(-)deprenyl prolongs life in aged male rats', *Life Sciences,* 47:415-420.

Milgram, NW, Ivy, GO, Head, E, *et al.* (1993), 'The effect of L-deprenyl on behavior, cognitive function, and biogenic amines in the dog', *Neurochemical Research,* 18: 1211-1219.

Mizuno, Y, Kondo, T, Kuno, S, *et al.* (2010), 'Early addition of selegiline to L-Dopa treatment is beneficial for patients with Parkinson's disease', *Clinical Neuropharmacology*, 33:1-4.

Miyoshi, K (2001), 'Parkinson's disease'. *Nippon Rinsho,* 59:1570-1573.

Monteverde, A, Gnemmi, P, Rossi, F, *et al.* (1990), 'Selegiline in the treatment of mild to moderate Alzheimer-type dementia', *Clinical Therapeutics,* 12:315-322.

Myttyla, VV, Sotaniemi, KA, Vourinen, JA, *et al.* (1992), 'Selegiline as initial treatment in *de novo* parkinsonian patiens', *Neurology*, 42:339-343.

Nguyen, TV & Juorio, AV (1989), 'Binding sites for brain trace amines', *Cellular and Molecular Neurobiology*, 9:297-311.

Nguyen, TV, Paterson, IA, Juorio, AV, *et al.* (1989), 'Tryptamine receptors: neurochemical and electrophysiological evidence for postsynaptic and functional binding sites', *Brain Research*, 476:85-93.

Nies, A, Robinson, DS, Davis, JM, *et al.* (1973), 'Changes in monoamine oxidase with aging', In: C Eisdorfer, WE Fann (Eds), *Psychopharmacology of aging, Advances in Behavioral Biology*, Plenum Press, New York, pp 41-54.

Nussbaum, RL & Ellis, CE (2003), 'Alzheimer's disease and Parkinson's disease', *New England Journal of Medicine*, 348:1356-1364.

Ohta, K, Ohta, M, Mizuta, I, *et al.* (2002), 'The novel catecholaminergic and serotonergic activity enhancer *R*-(-)-1-(benzofuran-2-yl)-2-propylaminopentane up-regulates neurotrophic factor synthesis in mouse astrocytes', *Neuroscience Letters,* 328:205-208.

Olanow, CW & Rascol, O (2010), 'The delayed-start study in Parkinson disease: can't satisfy everyone', *Neurology,* 74: 1149-1150.

Olanow, CW, Godbold, JH, Koller, W (1996), 'Effect of adding selegiline to levodopa in early, mild Parkinson's disease. Patients taking selegiline may have received more levodopa than necessary', *British Medical Journal,* 312:702-703.

Palhagen, S, Heinonen, EH, Hägglund, J, *et al.* (1998), 'Selegiline delays the onset of disability in *de novo* parkinsonian patients', Swedish Parkinson Study Group. *Neurology,* 51: 520-525.

Parkinson Study Group (1989), 'Effect of (-)deprenyl on the progression disability in early Parkinson's disease', *New England Journal of Medicine,* 321:1364-1371.

Parkinson Study Group (1993), 'Effect to tocopherol and (-)deprenyl on the progression of disability in early Parkinson's disease', *New England Journal of Medicine,* 328:176-183.

Parkinson Study Group (1996), 'Impact of deprenyl and tocopherol treatment of Parkinson's disease in DATATOP patients requiring levodopa', *Annals of Neurology,* 39:37-45.

Parkinson Study Group (2002), 'A controlled trial of rasagiline in early Parkinson disease: the TEMPO study', *Archives of Neurology,* 59: 1937-1943.

Piccinin, GL, Finali, G, Piccirilli, M (1990), 'Neuropsychological effects of L-deprenyl in Alzheimer's type dementia', *Clinical Neuropharmacology,* 13: 147-163.

Ponto, LL & Schultz, SK (2003), 'Ginkgo biloba extract: review of CNS effects', *Annals of Clinical Psychiatry,* 15:109-119.

Premont, RT, Gainetdinov, RR, Caron, MG (2001), 'Following the trace of elusive amines', *Proceedings of the Natural Academy of Sciences USA,* 98:9474-9475.

Quitkin, RT, Liebowitz, MR, Stewart, JW, *et al.* (1984), 'L-Deprenyl in atypical depression', *Archives of General Psychiatry,* 41:777-781.

Rapaport, MH & Thase, ME (2007), 'Translating the evidence on atypical depression into clinical practice', *Journal of Clinical Psychiatry,* 68: e11.

Ricci, A, Mancini, M, Strocchi, P, *et al.* (1992), 'Deficits in cholinergic neurotransmission markers induced by ethylcholine mustard aziridium (AF64A) in the rat hippocampus: sensitivity to treatment with the monoamine oxidase-B inhibitor L-deprenyl,' *Drug Experimental Clinical Research,* 18:163-171.

Riederer, P & Wuketich, S (1976), 'Time course of nigrostriatal degeneration in Parkinson's disease', *Journal Neural Transmission,* 38:277-301.

Riekkinen, PJ, Koivisto, K, Helkala, EL, *et al.* (1994), 'Long-term, double-blind trial of selegiline in Alzheimer's disease', *Neurobiology of Aging,* 15 (Suppl 1): S67.

Rinne, JO, Röyttä, M, Paljärvi, L, *et al.* (1991), 'Selegiline (deprenyl) treatment and death of nigral neurons in Parkinson's disease', *Neurology,* 41:859-861.

Ritter, JL & Alexander, B (1997), 'Retrospective study of selegiline-antidepressant drug interactions and a review of the literature', *Annals of Clinical Psychiarty,* 9:7-13.

Robinson, DS, Davis, JM, Nies, A, *et al.* (1971), 'Relation of sex and aging to monoamine oxidase activity of human brain, plasma and platelets', *Archives of General Psychiatry,* 24:536-539.

Robinson, DS, Davis, JM, Nies, A, *et al.* (1972), 'Aging, monoamines, and monoamine oxidase levels', *The Lancet,* i:290-291.

Robottom, BJ (2011), 'Efficacy, safety, and patient preference of monoamine oxidase B inhibitors in the treatment of Parkinson's disease', *Patient Preference and Adherence,* 5: 57-64.

Ruehl, WW, Bruyette, DS, DePaoli, A, *et al.* (1995), 'Canine cognitive dysfunction as a model for human age-related cognitive decline, dementia and Alzheimer's disease: clinical presentation, cognitive testing, pathology and response to l-deprenyl therapy', *Progress in Brain Research,* 106: 217-225.

Ruehl, WW, Entriken, TL, Muggenberg, BA, *et al.* (1997), 'Treatment with L-deprenyl prolongs life in elderly dogs', *Life Sciences,* 61:1037-1044.

Saavedra, JM (1974), 'Enzymatic isotopic assay for and presence of beta-phyenylathylamine in brain', *Journal of Neurochemistry,* 22:211-216.

Saavedra, JM (1989), 'Catecholamines II', In: U Trendelenburg, N Weiner (Eds), *Handbook experimental pharmacology,* Springer-Verlag, New York, pp. 181-201.

Sabelli, HC & Javaid, JI (1995), 'Phenylethylamine modulation of affect: therapeutic and diagnostic implication', *Journal of Neurophsychiatry and Clinical Neuroscience,* 7:6-14.

Sabelli, HC & Mosnaim, AD (1974), 'Phenylethylamine hypothesis of affective behavior', *American Journal of Psychiat*ry, 131:695-699.

Sabelli, HC, Fawcett, J, Gusovsky, F, *et al.* (1986), 'Clinical studies on the phenylethylamine hypothesis of affective disorder: urine and blood phenylacetic acid and phenylalanine dietary supplements', *Clinical Psychiatry,* 47:66-70.

Samuele, A, Mangiagalli, A, Armentero M, *et al.* (2005), 'Oxidative stress and pro-apoptotic conditions in a rodent model of Wilson's disease', *Biochimica et Biophysica Acta,* 1741:325-330.

Sandler, M, Glover, V, Ashford, A, *et al.* (1978), 'Absence of "cheese effect" during deprenyl therapy: some recent studies', *Journal Neural Transmission,* 43:209-215.

Sano, M, Ernesto, C, Thomas, RG, *et al.* (1997), 'A controlled trial of selegiline, alpha-tocopherol, or both as treatment for Alzheimer's disease', *New England Journal of Medicine,* 336:1216-1222.

Satoi, M, Matsuishi, T, Yamada, S, *et al.* (2000), 'Decreased cerebrosbinal fluid levels of beta-phenylethylamine in patients with Rett snydrome', *Annals of Neurology,* 47:801-803.

Schneider, LS, Olin, JT, Pavluczyk, S (1993), 'A double-blind cross-over pilot study of l-deprenyl (selegiline) combined with cholinesterase inhibitor in Alzheimer's disease', *American Journal of Psychiatry,* 150:321-323.

Schumacher, M, Weil-Engerer, S, Liere, P, *et al.* (2003), 'Steroid hormones and neurosteroids in normal and pathological aging of the nervous system', *Progress in Neurobiology,* 71:3-29.

Selkoe, DJ (2000), 'Toward a comprehensive theory for Alzheimer's disease. Hypothesis: Alzheimer's disease is caused by the cerebral accumulation and cytotoxicity of amyloid beta-protein', *Annals New York Academy of Sciences,* 924:17-25.

Shih, JC (1979), 'Monoamine oxidase in aging human brain', In: TP Singer, RW Korff, DL Murphy (Eds), *Monoamine oxidase: structure, function and altered functions.* Academic Press, New York, pp. 413-421.

Shimazu, S & Miklya, I (2004), 'Pharmacological studies with endogenous enhancer substances: β-phenylethyamine, tryptamine, and their synthetic derivatives', *Progress in Neuro-Psychopharmacology and Biological Psychiatry,* 28:421-427.

Shimazu, S, Tanigawa, A, Sato N, *et al.* (2003), 'Enhancer substances: Selegiline and *R*-(-)-1-(benzofuran-2-yl)-2-propylaminopentane, [(-)-BPAP] enhance the neurotrophic factor synthesis on cultured mouse astrocytes', *Life Sciences,* 72:2785-2792.

Shoulson, I (1998), 'DATATOP: a decade of neuroprotective inquiry. Parkinson Study Group. Deprenyl And Tocopherol Antioxidative Therapy Of Parkinsonism', *Annals Neurology,* 44 (3 Suppl 1): S160-166.

Stewart, JW (2007), 'Treating depression with atypical features', *Journal of Clinical Psychiatry*, 68 (Suppl 3): 25-29.

Stoll, S, Hafner, U, Kranzlin, B, Muller, WE (1997), 'Chronic treatment of Syrian hamsters with low-dose selegiline increases life span in females but not males', *Neurobiology of Aging*, 18:205-211.

Strolin Benedetti, M & Keane, PE (1980), 'Differential changes in monoamine oxidase A and B activity in the aging brain', *Journal of Neurochemistry*, 35:1026-1032.

Student, AK & Edwards, DJ (1977), 'Subcellular localization of types A and B monoamine oxidase in rat brain', *Biochemical Pharmacology*, 26:2337-2342.

Sunderland, T, Molchan, S, Lawlor, B, *et al.* (1992), 'A strategy of "combination chemotherapy" in Alzheimer's disease: rationale and preliminary results with physostigmin and deprenyl', *International Psychogeriatrics*, 4:291-308.

Tanner, CM & Goldmann, SM (1996), 'Epidemiology of Parkinson's disease', *Neurologic Clinic*, 14:317-335.

Tariot, PN, Cohen, RM, Sunderland, T, *et al.* (1987), 'L-(-)Deprenyl in Alzheimer's disease', *Archives of General Psychiatry*, 44:427-433.

Tariot, PN, Goldstein, B, Podgorski, CA, *et al.* (1998), 'Short-term administration of selegiline for mild-to-moderate dementia of the Alzheimer's type A', *Journal of Geriatric Psychiatry*, 6: 145-154.

Tatton. WG, Ju. WY, Holland. DP, *et al.* (1994), '(-)-Deprenyl reduces PC12 cell apoptosis by inducing new protein synthesis', *Journal of Neurochemisry*, 63:1572-1575.

Tatton, WG, Ansari, K, Yu W, *et al.* (1995), 'Selegiline induces "trophic-like" rescue of dying neurons without MAO inhibition', *Advances in Experimental Medicine and Biology*, 363:15-16.

Tetrud, JW & Langston, JW (1989), 'The effect of (-)deprenyl (selegiline) on the natural history of Parkinson's disease', *Science*, 245:519-522.

Thomas, T (2000), 'Monoamine oxidase-B inhibitors in the treatment of Alzheimer's disease', *Neurobiology of Aging*, 21:343-348.

Tom, T & Cummings, JL (1998), 'Depression in Parkinson's disease. Pharmacological characteristics and treatment', *Drugs & Aging*, 12:55-74.

Tong, J, Hornykiewicz, O, Kish, SJ (2006), 'Inverse relationship between brain noradrenaline level and dopamine loss in Parkinson Disease', *Archives of Neurology*, 63: 1724-1728.

Tóth, V, Kummert, M, Sugár, J, Knoll, J (1992), 'A procedure for measuring neuromelanin in neurocytes by a TV-image analyser', *Mechanisms of Ageing and Development*, 63:215-221.

Tringer, L, Haits, G, Varga, E (1971), 'The effect of (-)E-250, (-)L-phenyl-isopropylmethyl-propinyl-amine HCl, in depression', In: G Leszkovszky (Ed), *V. Conferentia Hungarica pro Therapia et Investigatione in Pharmacologia*, Akadémiai Kiadó (Publishing House of the Hungarian Academy of Sciences), Budapest, pp. 111-114.

Trivedy, MH, Rush, AJ, Wisniewski, SR, *et al.* (2006), 'Evaluation of outcomes with citalopram for depression using measurement-based care in STAR*D: implications for clinical practice', *American Journal of Psychiatry*, 163: 28-40.

Tsunekawa, H, Noda, Y, Mouri, A, *et al.* (2008), 'Synergistic effects of selegiline and donepezil on cognitive impairment induced by amyloid beta (25-35)', *Behavioral Brain Research*, 190: 224-232.

Usdin, E & Sandler, M (Eds) (1976), *'Trace amines and the brain'*, Marcel Dekker, NewYork

Varga, E (1965), 'Vorläufiger Bericht über die Wirkung des Präparats E-250 (phenyl-isopropyl-methyl-propinylamine-chlorhydrat)', In: B Dumbovich (Ed), *III. Conferentia Hungarica pro Therapia et Investigatione in Pharmacologia*, Akadémiai Kiadó (Publishing House of the Hungarian Academy of Sciences), Budapest, pp. 197-201.

Varga, E & Tringer, L (1967), 'Clinical trial of a new type of promptly acting psychoenergetic agent (phenyl-isopropylmethyl-propinylamine HCl, E-250)', *Acta Medica Hungarica*, 23:289-295.

Walker, SE, Shulman, KI, Tailor, SA, *et al.* (1996), 'Tyramine content of previously restricted foods in monoamine oxidase inhibitor diets', *Journal of Clinical Psychopharmacology*, 16:383-388.

Waters, CH (1994), 'Fluoxetine and selegiline – lack of significant interaction', *Canadian Journal of Neurological Sciences*, 21: 259-261.

Wecker, L, James, S, Copeland, N, *et al.* (2003), 'Transdermal selegiline: targeted effects on monoamine oxidases in the brain', *Biological Psychiatry*, 54:1099-1104.

Wilcock, GK, Birks, J, Whitehead, A, *et al.* (2002), 'The effect of selegiline in the treatment of people with Alzheimer's disease: a meta-analysis of published trials', *International Journal of Geriatric Psychiatry*, 17: 175-183.

Wilner, J, LeFevre, HF, Costa, E (1974), 'Assay by multiple ion detection of phenylethylamine and phenylethanolamine in rat brain', *Journal of Neurochemistry*, 23:857-859.

Zarow, C, Lynnes, SA, Mortimer, JA, Chui, HC (2003), 'Neuronal loss is greater in the locus coeruleus than nucleus basalis and substantia nigra in Alzheimer and Parkinson disease', *Archives of Neurology,* 60:337-341.

Zeller, EA, Barsky, J, Fouts, JE, *et al.* (1952), 'Influence of isonicotinic acid hydrazide (INH) and 1-isonicotinic 2-isopropylhydrazide (IIH) on bacterial and mammalian enzymes', *Experientia*, 8:349-350.

Zesiewicz, TA, Gold, M, Chari, G, *et al.* (1999), 'Current issues in depression in Parkinson's disease', *American Journal of Geriatric Psychiatry*, 7:110-118.

Zhao, YJ, Wee, HL, Au, WL, *et al.* (2011), 'Selegiline use is associated with a slower progression in early Parkinson's disease as evaluated by Hoehn and Yahr Stage transition times', *Parkinsonism & Related Disorders*, 17: 194-197.

Yen, TT & Knoll, J (1992), 'Extension of lifespan in mice treated with Dinh lang (Policias fruticosum L.) and (-)deprenyl', *Acta Physiologica Hungarica*, 79: 119-124.

Yen, TT, Dallo, J, Knoll, J (1982), 'The aphrodisiac effect of low doses of (-)deprenyl in male rats', *Polish Journal of Pharmacology & Pharmacy*, 34: 303-308.

Youdim, MB (1980), 'Monoamine oxidase inhibitors as anti-depressant drugs and as adjuct to L-dopa therapy of Parkinson's disease', *Journal Neural Transmission Suppl,* 16:157-161.

APPENDIX

CHRONOLOGY OF THE MILESTONES IN DEPRENYL (D) RESEARCH

D was created in the 1960s, in the midst of the golden era when within less than 20 years the development of crucially new families of important pharmacological agents, monoamine oxidase (MAO) inhibitors, phenothiazines, tricyclic antidepressants and uptake inhibitors, were brought into being. These discoveries led to the science of neuropsychopharmacology, which changed the principles of behavioral studies in a revolutionary manner and radically altered human attitudes toward derangements in psychic function. A volume edited in 1998 by TA Ban, D Healy and E Shorter, a retrospective of "The Rise of Psychopharmacology and the Story of CINP", stated that "Deprenyl, the first catecholaminergic activity enhancer" (pp. 91-94) belongs to the mainstream of drug development.

The most relevant interviews which informed the general reading public of deprenyl research include the following:

Medical Odyssey. Drug for Ills of the Old Is Drawing Deprenyl Attention after 30-year Struggle. Long Sidetracked, Helps with Parkinson's And Possibly Much More. Trading on Hungary's Jewels. By Michael Waldholz. An interview with Joseph Knoll. The Wall Street Journal. Vol. LXXII. No.31. Tuesday, November 27, 1990;

CBS Sixty Minutes (May, 1993);

David Healy: The Pharmacologists III. Arnold (2000). An interview with Joseph Knoll (Budapest). The Psychopharmacology of Life and Death, pp.81-110;

David J. Brown: Mavericks of Medicine. Conversations on the Frontiers of Medical Research. SmartPublications (2006). An interview with Joseph Knoll. Shattering the Barriers of Maximum Life Span, pp.137-147;

Knoll J interviewed by Ban TA, in *An Oral History of Neuropsychopharmacology - The First Fifty Years: Peer Interviews* (Thomas A. Ban editor), Volume 3 – "Neuropharmacology" (Fridoline Sulser, volume editor). Nashville: American College of Neuropsychopharmacology; 2011. pp. 297-328.

The last period of our structure activity relationship (SAR) study leading finally to the selection of dl-phenylisopropylmethyl-propinylamine • HCl (E-250), later named deprenyl, for development, coincided with the publication of a calamitous number of clinical reports in 1963 in Lancet I and II (Blackwell I. p.167, II. p.414; Davies II. p 587; Foster II. p.587; Maan II, p.639; Womack II, p.463). These reports gave accounts of the patients treated with MAO inhibitors (tranylcypromine, nialamide, pargyline) developed temporarily clinical symptoms similar to paroxysm produced by pheochromocytoma and this finding threw the MAO inhibitors into disrepute. Thus, the time was ripe and compelling for the development of new spectrum MAO inhibitors.

The aim of my planned SAR study was the development of a new stimulant that combines the psychostimulant effect of β-phenylethylamine (PEA), the physiologically highly important trace amine, with the psychoenergetic effect of the MAO inhibitors, the newly developed family of antidepressants. In compliance with this aim, the starting molecule of our SAR study was methamphetamine (MA), the long acting synthetic PEA-derivative. We synthetized new MA-derivatives and attached to each of the new, patentable molecules, a propargyl group to the nitrogen. This group binds covalently to the flavin in MAO and by this means blocks the enzyme irreversibly.

We found a couple of new PEA/MA-derivatives which acted like PEA and blocked MAO. I decided finally to select E-250 because of the unique behavior of this compound. E-250 significantly inhibited the pressor effect of amphetamine. This constituted a striking contrast to the effect of known MAO inhibitors which potentiated the pressor effect of amphetamine. This anomaly was shown in the first paper (Knoll *et al.*, 1965, Fig. **1**).

Further studies soon revealed that reasonable considerations shaped our SAR study and the selection of E-250 for development was a lucky decision.

*

The SAR study leading to the selection of D started in 1960, thus 52 years ago. In retrospect we can divide the 52 years into three periods.

THE FIRST REASERCH PERIOD: 1960-1978.

D achieved its place in research and therapy as the first selective inhibitor of MAO-B and we firmly believed that this unique effect of the drug is of primary therapeutic importance.

THE SECOND REASERCH PERIOD: 1979-1994

Accumulation of experimental data furnishing unequivocal evidence that D facilitates dopaminergic neurotransmission and the development of the concept that preventive D medication which facilitates dopaminergic and 'trace-aminergic' activity in the brain is a reasonable strategy to improve the quality of the postdevelopmental (aging) period of life. The performance of the two longevity studies showing that maintanence on D prolongs the life of rats significantly. Experimental evidence with the development of (-)-PPAP, the D-analoge free of MAO-B inhibitory potency of its parent compound, that the peculiar stimulation of the catecholaminergic neurons in the brain by D is unrelated to the selective inhibition of B-type MAO. The development of the method that ensured to get convincing evidence for the operation of the enhancer regulation in the life-important catecholaminergic and serotonergic neuronal systems in the brain stem.

THE THIRD REASERCH PERIOD: 1995-2011

Attention focused on the enhancer-regulation in the catecholaminergic and serotonergic neurons in the brain. The proof that PEA is a natural catecholaminergic activity enhancer (CAE) substance and in high concentration only a releaser of catecholamines from their interneuronal pools. Evidence that D inhibits MAO-B activity in high doses only and is primarily a synthetic PEA-derived selective CAE substance devoid of the catecholamine-releasing property of the parent compound. The proof that D is almost ineffective on the serotonergic neurons when compared to the dose in which it exerts its CAE effect. The development of R-(-)-1-(benzofuran-2yl)-2-propylaminopentane, (-)-BPAP (B), a highly potent serotonergic activity enhancer compound and a hundred times more potent CAE substance than D.

The following data provides evidence of the still undiminished international interest in D-research.

E-250/D/Selegiline(S) papers published since 1964. From 1978 until 2011 the S/D papers recorded in PubMed were considered.

Research Periods	Total Number of Published Papers	Average/Year
1964-1978	51	3.4
1979-1994	1010	63.1
1995-2011	1461	85.9

D is still used in research as the international reference compound to block B-type MAO selectively. As a therapeutic agent D, used to treat Parkinson's disease, Alzheimer's disease and major depressive disease, is registered in 63 countries, and marketed world-wide under more than 100 trade-names.

THE FIRST RESEARCH PERIOD: 1960-1978

ELABORATION OF THE WORK	THE RESULTS	THE FIRST PUBLICATION (S) OF THE RESULTS
1960-1965	***The structure activity relationship (SAR) study and the selection of E-250 (later named deprenyl) for further development.*** The chemical part of the SAR study was performed in collaboration with a group of chemists in Chinoin Pharmaceutical Company (Budapest) led by Zoltan Ecsery. It is mentioned already in the discussion of the first publication that "Preliminary investigation (E. Varga, personal communication) indicated that E-250 is highly active in cases of depression" (Knoll *et al.*, 1965, p.163).	Knoll J, Ecsery Z, Kelemen K, Nievel J, Knoll B (1964) (in Hungarian) Knoll J, Ecseri Z, Kelemen K, Nievel J, Knoll B (1965) (in English)
1964-1967	*The first clinical study with D.* A preliminary note on the promising results of the running clinical trial with (±)-E-250 in depressed patients. The first paper showing that (±)-E-250 is an efficient prompt acting antidepressant.	Varga E (1965) (in German) Varga E & Tringer L (1967)
1966-1967	The analysis showing that (-)-E-250 is a more potent MAO inhibitor than (+)-E-250.	Magyar K, Vizi ES, Ecseri Z, Knoll J (1967)
1967	***(-)-E-250 was selected for further development.***	
1967-1968	The exact experimental analysis showing that (-)-E-250 is a unique MAO inhibitor which does not potentiate the catecholamine-releasing effect of tyramine, thus the compound is free of the cheese effect. Varga E showed in an unpublished pilot study that in harmony with our findings in animal experiments (-)-E-250 is also free of the cheese effect in humans. This finding was cited in the discussion of our paper: "Even provocative cheese consumption (Varga, personal communication) failed to produce headache or hypertensive crisis" (p.111)	Knoll J, Vizi ES, Somogyi G (1968)
1968-1971	The first report on the clinical trial with (-)-E-250 in depressed patients showing its significant antidepressant effect.	Tringer L, Haits G, Varga E (1971)
1970-1972	*The discovery that (-)-deprenyl (D) is a **selective inhibitor of B-type MAO**. Lecture by Knoll J, First Symposium on MAO in Cagliary (Italy) (1971) First published paper demonstrating in detail that D is a selective inhibitor of B-type of MAO. The paper became a Citation Classic in 1982.	Knoll J & Magyar K (1972)

1974-1976	Analysis of the pharmacological effects of selective MAO inhibitors. The simultaneous oxidation of labeled monoamines in the presence and absence of selective MAO inhibitors (D and clorgyline) by rat liver and brain mitochondrial MAO was studied with double-labeling technique. Striking differences in the effect of D and clorgyline on isolated organs was demonstrated. The therapeutic aspect of the selective inhibitors was evaluated. Lecture at the Second International Symposium on MAO. CIBA Foundation Symposium. London (1975)	Knoll, J (1976)
1976-1978	The first study showing the peculiar pharmacological spectrum of D from new aspects. It was shown that D was unique in inhibiting tyramine uptake in a battery of tests. D was found to inhibit the release of acetylcholine in isolated striatal slices of the rat, owing to its blocking effect on the uptake of dopamine. *The drug protects the nigrostriatal dopaminergic neurons from the toxic effect of 6-hydroxy-dopamine. First proof of the* **neuroprotective** *effect of D.*	Knoll J (1978)
1977-1978	*Two papers published in the same year, produced sufficient proof that D is free of the cheese effect in humans.* After pretreatment with D parkinsonian volunteers who received levodopa or levodopa+carbidopa suffered no adverse pressor reaction after challenge with oral tyramine in considerably greater amounts than those likely to be encountered in a normal diet.	Elsworth JD, Glover V, Reynolds GP, Sandler M, Less AJ, Phuapradit P, Shaw KM, Stern GM, Kumar P (1978) Sandler M, Glover V, Ashford A, Stern GM (1978)
1975-1982	The first clinical trial proving that with the concurrent administration of levodopa with D the levodopa sparing effect is achieved in patients without signs of significant hypertensive reactions. *This study initiated and the following Lancet Editorial enhanced the world-wide use of D in Parkinson's disease.*	Birkmayer W, Riederer P, Ambrozi L, Youdim MBH (1977) Lancet Editorial (1982)
1978-1980	The first confirmation of the significant antidepressant effect of D in major depressive disease.	Mann JJ, Gershon S (1980)

THE SECOND RESEARCH PERIOD: 1979-1994

ELABORATION OF THE WORK	THE RESULTS	THE FIRST PUBLICATION (S) OF THE RESULTS
1979-1982	Accumulation of experimental data furnishing unequivocal evidence that D facilitates dopaminergic neurotransmission and the development of the concept that preventive D medication which facilitates dopaminergic and 'trace-aminergic' activity in the brain is a reasonable strategy to improve the quality of life in the latter decades. The restitution and longterm maintenance of full scale sexual activity in aged male rats continuously treated with D was demonstrated as an experimental model in support of the view that the longterm administration of small doses of D may improve the quality of life in the declining years. Lecture at the Strategy in Drug Research IUPAC-IUPHAR Symposium, (1981) Noordwijkerhout, The Netherlands	Knoll J (1982)
1982-1985	Final proof of the facilitation of dopaminergic activity by D and experimental evidence that this effect is unrelated to the inhibition of B-type MAO. Lecture presented at the 7th European Symposium on Basic Research in Gerontology, (1983) Budapest (Hungary)	Knoll J (1985)
1977-1985	In an open, uncontrolled study the long term (9 years) effect of treatment with Madopar alone (n=377) or in combination with D (n=564) have been compared in parkinsonian patents. The survival analysis revealed a significant increase of life expectancy in Madopar+D group regardless of the fact whether or not the significant demographic differences between the two groups were taken into account.	Birkmayer W, Knoll J, Riederer P, Youdim MBH, Hars V, Marton V (1985)
1986-1987	Two clinical studies, published independently from each other in the same year, described the beneficial effect of D-treatment in Alzheimer's disease.	Martini E, Pataky I, Szilágyi K, Venter V (1987) Tariot PN, Cohen RM, Sunderland T, Newhouse PA, Yount D, Mellow AM (1987)
1985-1988	*The first longevity study with D on Wistar-Logan rats starting with 2-year old males.* The proof that the maintenance of aged male rats on D restored full scale sexual activity and prolonged their life significantly. The longest living rat in the saline-treated	Knoll J (1988) Knoll J, Dalló J, Yen TT (1989)

	group lived 164 weeks. The average lifespan of the group was 147.05±0.56 weeks. The shortest living animal in the D-treated group lived 171 weeks and the longest living rat died during the 226th week of its life. The average lifespan was 197.98±2.36 weeks, *i.e.* higher than the estimated maximum age of death in this robust strain of rats (182 weeks). This was the first instance in which medicated members of a species lived beyond the estimated lifespan maximum. The evidence of the outstanding learning performance of 8-month-old sexually active rats compared to their sexually inactive peers.	
1987-1989	*First proof that D-treatment enhances significantly the activity of superoxide dismutase (SOD) in the striatum of both male and female rats.* The justness of the conclusion that the increased SOD activity was just a sign of D-induced enhanced activity of the nigrostriatal dopaminergic neurons was demonstrated by measuring SOD activity in the cerebellum which, as expected, remained unchanged in D-treated rats.	Knoll J (1988) Knoll J (1989)
1989-1990	First confirmation that D prolongs the life of rats. The longevity study was performed on the short living Fischer F-344 strain of rats.	Milgram MW, Racine RJ, Nellis P, Mendoca A, Ivy GO (1990)
1990-1991	*First confirmation that D enhances scavenger function in the striatum.* Daily sc. injection of D for 3 weeks in young male rats caused a threefold increased in SOD activity in the striatum of the brain compared with the value in saline-injected control rats. It was shown that the activity of catalase (but not of glutathion peroxidase) was also significantly increased by D-treatment.	Carrillo MC, Kanai S, Nokubo M, Kitani K (1991)
1987-1989	In the DATATOP multicenter clinical trial (USA, Canada) in 23 University Institutions, the ability of D and tocopherol, antioxidant agents that act through complementary mechanisms were studied, expecting to delay the onset of disability necessitating levodopa therapy (the primary end point) in patients with early, untreated Parkinson's disease. Eight hundred subjects were randomly assigned in a two-by-two factorial design to receive D, tocopherol, a combination of both drugs, or placebo, and were followed up to determine the frequency of development to the end point. *The DATATOP study proved that the treatment of de novo parkinsonians with D (selegiline) has a unique beneficial influence on the natural history of Parkinson's*	Tetrud JW, Langston JW (1989) Parkinson Study Group (1989)

	disease. D-treatment delayed significantly the need for levodopa therapy. *The study also revaled that in contrast to the expectation of the authors, α-tocopherol was devoid of the beneficial effect of D.* The reason of this difference between D and α-tocopherol was shown by us later. D is enhancing the impulse propagation mediated release of dopamine (CAE effect) whereas α-tocopherol is in this respect ineffective (Miklya I, Knoll B, Knoll J, 2003). The DATATOP multicenter trial proved the justness of our conclusion that the CAE effect of D is responsible for the beneficial effect of the drug.	
1990-1999	The finding of the Parkinson Study Group that it is reasonable to start treatment of *de novo* Parkinson's disease with D in order to delay the onset of disability associated with early, otherwise untreated Parkinson's disease, was confirmed in French, Finnish, Swedish, and Norwegian-Danish multicenter studies.	Allain H, Gougnard J, Naukirek HC (1991) Myttyla VV, Sotaniemi KA, Vourinen JA, Heinonen EH (1992) Palhagen, S, Heinonen, EH, Hägglund, J, Kaugesaar T, Kontants H, Mäki-Ikola O, Palm R, Turunen J (1998) Larsen JP, Boas J, Erdal JE (1999)
1990-1992	*A SAR study aiming to develop a D-analog free of the MAO-B inhibitory potency.* The selection of 1-phenyl-2-propylaminopentane [(-)-PPAP], a D-analog which differs from D by containing instead of the propargyl-group a propyl-group, thus is free of the MAO-B inhibitory potency. The proof that (-)-PPAP is as potent as D as a CNS stimulant. The chemical part of the SAR study was performed with a group of chemist in Chinoin Pharmaceutical Company (Budapest) led by Zoltan Török. *The development of (-)-PPAP was direct proof that the peculiar stimulation of the catecholaminergic neurons in the brain by D is unrelated to the inhibition of B-type MAO.*	Knoll J, Knoll B, Török Z, Timár J, Yasar S (1992a)
1990-1992	Morphological evidence in rats that D-treatment prevents aging-related pigment changes in the substantia nigra. With the aid of TV-image analysis, the number, the area and the density features of melanin granules in neurocytes of the substantia nigra in a group of 3-month-old naïve male rats and in a 21-month-old group of male rats treated for 18 months with saline and D respectively, were determined.	Knoll, J, Tóth, V, Kummert, M, Sugár, J (1992b)

1990-1994	*The second longevity study starting with 28-week-old Wistar-Logan male rats.*	Knoll J, Yen TT, Miklya I (1994)
	Out of 1600 sexually inexperienced rats the 94 sexually inactive (low performing, LP) and the 99 most sexually active (high performing, HP) rats were selected. The LP rats died significantly earlier than their HP peers and D-treatment eliminated this difference.	
	The rats were treated from 8th month of their life three times a week with 0.25 mg/kg D and saline, respectively, until they died. The salt-treated LP rats (n=44) never displayed ejaculations and lived 134.58±2.29 weeks, their D-treated peers (n=48) became sexually active and lived 152.54±1.36 weeks. The salt-treated HP rats (n=49) lived 151.24±1.36 weeks, their D-treated peers (n=50) lived 185.30±1.96 weeks and out of the 50 rats 17 lived longer than the estimated technical lifespan (TLS).	
	This longevity study was further unequivocal experimental evidence that D-treatment prolongs the life of rats significantly.	
1992-1994	First proof that D reduces PC12 cell apoptosis by inducing new protein synthesis.	Tatton WG, Ju WY, Holland DP, Tai C, Kwan M (1994)
1992-1994	The HPLC method with electrochemical detection allowed measuring exactly the release of dopamine from the striatum, tuberculum olfactorium and substantia nigra, the release of norepinephrine from the locus coeruleus, and the release of serotonin from the raphe, in the amounts released from freshly excised brain tissue. *The method ensured to get convincing evidence for the operation of the enhancer regulation in the life-important catecholamin-ergic and serotonergic neuronal systems in the brain stem.*	Knoll J & Miklya I (1994)
1993-1994	Confirmation of the prolonged lifespan of mice on D.	Freisleben, HJ, Lehr, F, Fuchs, J (1994)

THE THIRD RESEARCH PERIOD: 1995-2011

ELABORATION OF THE WORK	THE RESULTS	THE FIRST PUBLICATION (S) OF THE RESULTS
1994-1995	Demonstration that in both male and female rats the resting release of transmitters from brain catecholaminergic and serotonergic neurons during the period from weaning until the end of the second month of age, *i.e.* during the crucial developmental phase of their life, was significantly higher than either before or after that period, signalling the transition from the developmental to the post-developmental (aging) phase of life. *This finding showed that on one hand, sexual hormones might play the main role in terminating the enhanced catecholaminergic activity characteristic to the post-weaning period, since the enhancer regulation is terminated at the end of the second month of age when the rats arrive to sexual maturity. On the other hand, this finding clearly indicated that safe and effective measures are needed to maintain the catecholaminergic system at a higher activity level during the post-developmental, downhill period of life.*	Knoll J & Miklya I (1995)
1995-1996	Demonstration that β-phenylethylamine (PEA), the physiologically highly important stimulatory trace-amine in the brain, known as a classic releaser of catecholamines from their intraneuronal pools, is a mixed acting sympathomimetic. *PEA is in low concentration devoid of the releasing property and acts as a natural CAE substance, a selective enhancer of the impulse propagation mediated release of catecholamines.*	Knoll, J, Miklya, I, Knoll, B, Markó, R, Rácz, D (1996c)
1995-1996	*Demonstration that D and (-)-PPAP, the D-derivative free of MAO-B inhibitory potency, are unique PEA-derivatives which lost the ability of PEA to induce the continuous release of catecholamines from intraneuronal pools, but maintained the specific catecholaminergic activity enhancer (CAE) property of their parent compound.*	Knoll, J, Miklya, I, Knoll, B, Markó, R, Kelemen, K (1996a)
1995-1997	The first controlled trial of D (selegiline) as treatment for Alzheimer's disease.	Sano M, Ernesto C, Thomas RG, Klauber MR, Schafer K, Grundman M, Woodbury P, Growdon J, Cotman CW, Pfeiffer E, Schneider LS, Thal LJ (1997)

1987-1999	First proofs for the protective effect of enhancer substances (D, B) against various neurotoxins.	
	D protects against MPTP toxicity.	Cohen G, Pasik P, Cohen B, Leist A, Mitileneou C, Yahr MD (1984) Heikkila, RE, Hess, A, Duvoisin, RC (1985)
	D-treatment protects the dopaminergic neurons from the toxic effect of 6-OH-dopamine (6-OHDA).	Knoll J, (1978, 1987) Hársing LG, Magyar K, Tekes K, Vizi ES, Knoll J (1979)
	D blocks DSP-4 toxicity.	Gibson CJ (1987)
	D prevents the neurotoxic effect of 5,6-dihydroxyserotonin.	Ebadi, M, Sharma, S, Shavali S, El Refaey H (2002)
	D protects against AF64A toxicity.	Ricci A, Mancini M, Strocchi P, Bongrani S, Bronzetti E (1992)
	B protects cultured hippocampal neurons from the toxic effect of β-amyloid$_{25-35}$.	Knoll J, Yoneda F, Knoll B, Ohde H, Miklya I (1999)
1996-1997	Confirmation of the lifespan prolonging effect of D on Syrian hamsters	Stoll, S, Hafner, U, Kranzlin, B, Muller, WE (1997)
	Treatment with D prolongs life in elderly dogs.	Ruehl WW, Entriken TL, Muggenberg BA, Bruyette DS, Griffith WG, Hahn FF (1997)
1998	The final analysis in support of the concept that D (selegiline) is a PEA derived *selective* CAE substance devoid of the side effect of its parent compound which in higher concentration elicits the continuous release of catecholamines from their intraneuronal pools. D exerts its CAE effect in concentrations below the ones needed to block MAO-B activity significantly.	Knoll J (1998)
1995-1999	***The development of R-(-)-1-(benzofuran-2-yl)-2-propylaminopentane [(-)-BPAP]*** (B) a tryptamine-derived selective enhancer of the impulse propagation mediated release of catecholamines and serotonin in the	Knoll J, Yoneda F, Knoll B, Ohde H, Miklya I (1999)

	brain. The chemical part of the SAR study was performed in collaboration with a group of chemists in Fujimoto Pharmaceutical Company (Osaka) led by Fumio Yoneda.	
1999	Prolongation of life with D in an experimental model of aging in Drosophila melanogaster.	Jordens RG, Berry MD, Gillott C, Boulton AA (1999)
1996-2000	*Demonstration that, in harmony with our expectation (Knoll & Miklya, 1995), sexual hormones terminated the significantly enhanced basic activity of the catecholaminergic and serotonergic neurons in the brain, characteristic to the post-weaning period, and brings back the enhancer regulation in these neurons to the pre-weaning lower level.* This exactly measurable qualitative change signals the transition from the pleasant but short developmental, uphill period of youthfulness, into the longer lasting, slowly decaying, post-developmental, downhill, aging period of life, irresistibly leading to death. The discovery of this mechanism clearly indicated that the aging-related, irresistible decay of the enhancer-regulation in the catecholaminergic neurons which play a leading role in the activation of the cortex, is a key important factor in brain aging. Thus, the maintenance of the activity of these neurons on a higher activity level during the postdevelopmental phase of life might significantly improve the quality of life in senescence.	Knoll, J, Miklya, I, Knoll, B, Dalló, J (2000)
2000-2005	*The final analysis that D is a unique anti-aging drug because it slows as a specific CAE substance the aging-related decay of the catecholaminergic system in the brain.* This conclusion is supported by the outcome of studies into the nature of the enhancer regulation in the catecholaminergic system, thus finding that this regulation is enhanced after weaning and sexual hormones bring back the regulation to the pre-weaning level. The results of the longevity studies with D argue definitely in favor of the concept that the aging of the brain starts as soon as sexual hormones terminate the enhanced catecholaminergic tone in the brain characteristic to the post-weaning, developmental, uphill period of life. Thus, sexual hormones elicit the transition of the developmental phase of life into the post-developmental, downhill (aging) period. The aging related slow decline of the enhancer regulation in the catecholaminergic system in the brain stem, the main activator of the cortex, is the prime factor of brain aging. The decay of the enhancer regulation in the most rapidly	Knoll J (2001, 2003, 2005)

	aging dopaminergic system is, for example, mainly responsible for the decline in learning ability and sexual activity with the passing of time.	
	The catecholaminergic system's ability to activate the higher brain centers sinks finally below a critical threshold and an emergency incident transpires, where a high level of activation is needed to survive and the CNS can no longer be activated to the required extent. This would explain why a common infection, a broken leg, or any other challenge easily surmountable given catecholaminergic machinery working at full capacity may cause death in old age. All in all, to keep the system *via* the administration of a small daily dose of a CAE substance (for example D) on a higher activity level, thus to fight against the physiological aging-related slow decay of this life-important system, improves the quality of life in senescence and prolongs life as shown by longevity studies performed with D. In conclusion, the enhancer substances are the first anti-aging compounds the safe prophylactic administration of which during the post-developmental, downhill period of life slows the physiological aging of the brain.	
1953-2005	***The enhancer regulation is now an integral part of the theory that tries to analyse the neurochemical basis of the drives (Knoll J, 2005).***	Knoll J (1969, 1994, 2001, 2003, 2005)
	The first attempt, based on the results of behavioral studies performed from 1953 until 1969, was summarized in a monograph (Knoll J, 1969). The second attempt, based on the results of the research period from 1969 until 2005, was summarized in a new monograph (Knoll J, 2005).	
	In behavioral studies 'drive' is the commonly used technical term to define the force that activates the mammalian organism. It is the inner urge that initiates a response, incites activity, and that represents a basic or instinctive need, such as the hunger drive, the sexual drive, and so on.	
	The neurochemical basis of both categories of drives - (a) the innate ones necessary for the survival of the individual and the species, and (b) the acquired ones for attaining an unlimited number of dispensable goals - is unknown. The brain mechanism that keeps the innate drives in action is presumably the less complicated part of the problem. The real crux of the issue seems to be the cortical mechanism that renders the acquisition of an unnatural urge possible.	
	Being familiar with a technical term we may occasionally have the erroneous impression of possessing full knowledge of the subject it connotes. For example: An eagle pounces upon a quiet, eating rabbit with lightning	

speed. The rabbit is given a split second to run for life. Common sense, practical explanation independent of specialized knowledge, is simple. Hunger drives the eagle and fear drives the rabbit. In reality, drive is just a useful description for the still unknown brain mechanism that activates the organism and keeps it in motion until the goal is reached.

For living beings with highly refined brain organization the cortex has absolute priority in maintaining the sophisticated integration between an apparently confusing network of cells, synchronizing them into a lucidly arranged, harmoniously operating system. For a highly refined organism, life means the operation of the integrative work of the brain, and natural death means the cessation of this function. This is clearly shown by the fact that cells of vital organs, including the brain, maintain vigorous activity for a short while even beyond the termination of the integrative work of the brain.

Enhancer regulation, primarily in the catecholaminergic neurons, keeps the telencephalon active and thus the system alive. The operation of the catecholaminergic system is comparable to an engine ignited once and for all in an early phase of development, and is signalled by the appearence of the EEG. Due to its enhancer regulation, the catecholaminergic system dynamically changes the activation of the cortex during lifetime according to need. Life is terminated because of the progressive decay of the efficiency of the catecholaminergic system during postdevelopmental lifespan until at some point, in an emergency situation, the integration of the parts in the highly sophisticated entity can no longer be maintained. Thus natural death, signalled by the disappearence of EEG, sets in (Knoll, 1994).

The catecholaminergic tone determines the three basic modes of brain activity. The system performs: (a) at its lowest possible level in the 'non-vigilant resting state' (sleeping); (b) at a steady low level in the 'vigilant resting state' (leisure); and (c) operates, according to the need, at a dynamically enhanced activity level in the 'active state' (exemplified by 'fight or flight' or goal-seeking-behavior).

Experimental evidence and theoretical considerations led to the conceptualization that an until recently unknown brain mechanism, the enhancer regulation in the brain, is primarily responsible for the innate drives, and a special form of it in the cortex is primarily responsible for the acquired drives. Furthermore, data supports the conclusion that age-related changes in the enhancer regulation of the catecholaminergic brain engine are primarily responsible for: (a) the youthful power of the mammals from weaning until sexual maturity; (b) the

	transition from the uphill period of life into postdevelopmental longevity; (c) the progressive decay of behavioral performances during the downhill period; (d) the transition from life to death. Finally, the data reinforce the proposal that prophylactic administration of a synthetic CAE substance during postdevelopmental life could significantly slow the unavoidable decay of behavioral performances, prolong life, and prevent or delay the onset of age-related neurodegenerative diseases, such as Parkinson's and Alzheimer's.	
2002-2003	B up-regulates neurotrophic factor synthesis in mouse astrocytes. But only the nonspecific enhancer effect of D and B is detectable on mouse astrocytes.	Ohta K, Ohta M, Mizuta I, Fujinami A, Shimazu S, Sato N, Yoneda F, Hayashi K, Kuno S (2002) Shimazu S, Tanigawa A, Sato N, Yoneda F, Hayashi K, Knoll J (2003)
2000-2006	The development of the selegiline transdermal system (STS). The first double blind, placebo-controlled, parallel group study in outpatients with STS. Emsam, the first transdermal antidepressant was registered in the USA in 2006.	Bodkin JA & Amsterdam JK (2002)
2001-2002	Proof that enhancer substances stimulate the enhancer-sensitive neurons in the brain in a peculiar manner. Two bell-shaped concentration effect curves characterize the effect. The one in the low pico-femtomolar level with a peak-effect at 10^{-13}-10^{-14}M concentration clearly demonstrates the existence of a specific form of the enhancer regulation; the second, in the micromolar range, with a peak effect 10^{-5}-10^{-6}M concentration shows the operation of an obviously non-specific form of the enhancer regulation in the enhancer-sensitive neurons.	Knoll J, Miklya I, Knoll B (2002a)
2001-2003	Due to its enhancer-effect B enhances the electrical stimulation induce release of [3H]-norepinephrine with the highly characteristic bi-modal, bell-shaped dose-effect relationship. We measured in this test in comparison to B the effect of drugs (desmethylimipramine, clorgyline, lazabemide, bromocryptine, pergolide, fluoxetin) used today clinically to stimulate the activity of the noradrenergic and/or dopaminergic and/or serotonergic neurons in the brain stem. None of the tested compounds shared with B the	Miklya I, Knoll J (2003)

	enhancer effect.	
2002-2003	In the DATATOP study the authors expected D to be efficient in their trial because of its MAO-B inhibitory effect. Their hypothesis was that the activity of MAO and the formation of free radicals predispose patients to nigral degeneration and contribute to the emergence and progression of Parkinson's disease. In accordance with their working hypothesis they expected that D, the MAO-inhibitor, and tocopherol, the antioxidant, and the combination of the two compounds will slow the clinical progress of the disease. They selected patients with early, untreated Parkinson's disease and measured the delay in the onset of disability necessitating levodopa therapy. In contrast to their expectation the study revealed that the risk of reaching the end of the trial was reduced by 57% for the subjects who received D, and these patients also had a significant reduction in their risk of having to give full time employment (Parkinson Study Group 1989). Tocopherol, however, was ineffective. The ineffectiveness was finally concluded following the course of changes (Parkinson Study Group 1992). *Since our studies convincingly proved that the observed beneficial effect of D in the DATATOP study must be related to its exactly demonstrated peculiar enhancer effect on the dopaminergic neurons, we compared the effect of D and tocopherol in our tests and, as expected, we found that tocopherol was devoid of an enhancer effect.*	Miklya I, Knoll B, Knoll J (2003a)
2010-	**We started on May 2010 our first longevity study on Wistar (Charles-River) male rats with D and B, treating the animals with low doses in which D and B exert their specific and nonspecific enhancer effect, respectively.** In the belief that the beneficial effects of D is related to the inhibition of MAO-B, we treated the rats in our earlier longevity studies with 0,25 mg/kg D. This is the lowest dose in which D blocks MAO-B activity in the brain completely. In this still running study we treat the rats with 0.001 and 0.1 mg/kg D, respectively. This is our first longevity study with B. We treat the rats with 0.0001 and 0.05 mg/kg B, respectively. Chapter 9 is summarizing our experiences with the rats in this still running longevity study to the end of the 18th month of their life. Since the running longevity experiment is the first analysis with low doses of D and B, respectively, the already observable differences in the dying out of the saline *versus* drug treated rats supports the opinion that the CAE effect is responsible for the well-known lifespan	

prolonging effect D and B acts in this respect like D.

CLOSING REMARKS

Since the catecholaminergic and serotonergic neurons in the brain stem play a leading role in the control of a lot of life important mechanisms, the discovery of the operation of the enhancer regulation in these neurons makes by itself the importance of this previously unknown regulation obvious. On the other hand, the finding that D is a selective CAE substance and practically ineffective on the serotonergic system, whereas B, a CAE substance much more potent than D, is even a more potent enhancer of the serotonergic neurons, clearly indicate that on a molecular level the enhancer regulation in the catecholaminergic and serotonergic neurons cannot be identical. There can be little doubt that we are at the very beginning to take the measure of the physiological role of the enhancer regulation in the brain. At present we just see the peak of an iceberg. It is reasonable to concentrate our efforts in the near future on the exploration of hitherto unknown enhancer-sensitive regulations in the mammalian brain. The fact that B exerts its specific enhancer effect in vivo in a dose as low as 0.0001 mg/kg and on cultured neurons in a concentration as low as 10^{-13}-10^{-14}M, means that we already possess a particularly suitable experimental tool for such studies.

Author Index

A

Adams SJ, see Bickford PC
Adham N, see Borowsky B
Agnoli A, 64, *93*
Ahlskog JE, 57, *93*
Aisen PS, see Lawlor BA
Albano C, see Loeb C
Alexander B, see Ritter JL
Alexopoulos GS, 74, *93*
Allain H, 54, *93*
Alzheimer A, 62
Amsterdam JD, 73, *93*; see Bodkin JA
Angst J, 71, *93*
Ansari K, see Tatton WG
Archer JR, 51, *93*
Armantero M, see Samuele A
Arttamankul S, see Bunzow JR
Ashford A, see Sandler M
Au WL, see Zhao YJ
Azzaro AJ, 73, *93*

B

Bakhshalizadeh S, 41, *93*
Ban TA, ii, 71, 107, *93*
Barbui C, see Cipriani A
Basak JM, see Kim J
Barsky J, see Zeller A
Berry MD, see Jordens MG
Bertler A, 46, *93*
Bickford PC, 51-52, *93*
Bierer LM, see Marin DB
Birkmayer W, 5, 53, 60, 87, *93*
Birks J, 64-65, *94*, see Wilcock GK
Blackwell B, 3, *94*
Blaschko H, xv-xvi, *94*
Blott LF, see Azzaro A
Boas J, see Larsen JP
Bodkin JA, 73, *94*
Borowsky B, 44, *94*
Boulton AA, 44, *94*; see Davis BA
Bovet D , 77, *94*; see Kelemen K
Bovet-Nitti F, see Bovet D
Boyson P, see Banasr M

Subject Index

A

Aging 42-53
- external appearance 42
- decrement of functions 42
- chronological age 42
- physiological age 42
- uphill period of life 26-29
- downhill period of life 26-29
- reparable biochemical lesions of brain aging
-- progressively developing dopaminergic and trace aminergic deficiency 45-47
-- enhanced MAO-B activity 44-45
Alzheimer's disease (AD) 62-68
- subtypes 62
- prevalence 63
- sex differences in incidence 63
- geographical differences in incidence 63
- genetic risk factors 63
- morphological changes 64-65
- therapy 64-68
Aβ(1-42) peptide (Abeta peptide) 66
- Aβ(25-35) fragment 38, 67-68, 85
Amphetamines iii, xv, 7-8, 10
- catecholamine releasing effect 13
Amitryptiline 71
Apolipoprotein E (APOE) protein 63
Atypical depression 69-74

B

(-)-BPAP [R-(-)-1-(benzofuran-2-yl)-2-propylaminopentane]
- enhancer effect 15-17, 78-79
-- specific enhancer effect 15
-- nonspecific enhancer effect 15
-- peculiar dose-dependency of the enhancer effect 17, 78-79
- longevity study 76-86
-- enhanced learning performance 81
-- prolongation of lifespan 82
- protects from the toxic effect of Aβ(25-35) peptide 38, 67-68
- upregulates neurotrophic factor synthesis 121
Bromocryptine 84, 122

C

Catatonic depression 70
Cheese effect 3-5, 71-72, 111
Clorgyline 84, 112, 127
Cognitive disfunction syndrome (CDS) 65-66
  - existence of Aβ plaques 65
  - (-)-deprenyl (Anipryl) for treatment in dogs 65
  - (-)-deprenyl (Selgian) for treatment in cats 66
Conditioned avoidance response (CAR) 77, 80
Cortical neurons, belonging to
  - Group 1 (untrained neurons) xii
  - Group 2 (extinguishable conditioned reflex, ECR) xii
  - Group 3 (inextinguishable conditioned reflex, ICR) xii
  - Group 4 (acquired drive) xii

D

DATATOP multicenter study of the Parkinson Study Group 53-57, 87-88, 114-115, 122-123
Dementia with Lewy bodies 62
(-)-Deprenyl (Selegiline) 3-14, 76-89, 107-115, 123
  - E250 (original code name) iii, xv, 4, 10, 107-108
  - selective MAO-B inhibitory effect 3-5
  - catecholaminergic activity enhancer (CAE) effect 6-16
  - tyramine inhibitory property 3-5
  - absence of catecholamine-releasing property 3-5
  - antiaging effect 40, 76-83
  - morphological evidence of antiaging effect 40-41, 115
  - enhanced production of neurotrophins (NGF, BDNF, GDNF) 37
  - longevity studies 17-20, 48-50, 76-86, 90, 112-114, 116
  - prolongs lifespan 51, 82, 113-114, 116-118
  -- beagle dogs 51, 118
  -- fly (Drosophyla melanogaster) 51, 118
  -- mice 51, 116
  -- rats
  --- Fischer 344 44, 51-52
  --- Wistar-Logan 20, 51, 113-114, 116
  --- Wistar (Charles River) 82
  -- Syrian hamster 51, 118
  - enhanced sexual activity 17-20,
  - enhanced learning performance 18-19, 80-81
  - enhances scavenger function 114
  - protects against neurotoxins 36-37, 118
  -- MPTP 36-37, 118
  -- 6OHDA 35-36, 118
  -- DSP4 37, 118

Selective serotonin reuptake inhibitors (SSRI) 53, 72
Selegiline, see (-)-deprenyl
Sexual hormones dampen enhancer regulation 29-33
Sexual activity in human males 47-48
Sexual activity (mounting, intromission, ejaculation) in male rats 49-50
Shuttle box 77
- method for measuring the specific and nonspecific enhancer effect of (-)-deprenyl and (-)-BPAP in vivo 78-79

T

Tacrine 63
Talent 21
Technical life span (TLS) xv, 25, 42, 76
Testosterone 29-33
- dampens enhancer regulation in the catecholaminergic and serotonergic neurons 30-33
Tetrabenazine 77-78, 84
α-Tocopherol 56-57, 64, 87, 115, 123
Trace-amines 43
Trace-amine (TA) receptors 44
Transition from life to death 23-25
Transition from uphill to downhill period of life 26-30
Tranylcypramine 108
Tricyclic antidepressants 107
Tryptamine 8-10
- enhancer effect 11-12
Tyramine 3-5, 73, 111-112
- role in "cheese effect" 3

U

Uphill period of life 23-30

V

Vascular dementia 62
Vitamin E: see α-Tocopherol

W

Weaning 24
- enhanced catecholaminergic and serotonergic activity after weaning 26-29

www.ingramcontent.com/pod-product-compliance
Lightning Source LLC
Chambersburg PA
CBHW041709210326
41598CB00007B/587